Pregnancy
The inside story

Joan Raphael-Leff, a practising psychoanalyst, is a
full member of the British Psycho-Analytical
Society and the International Psychoanalytical
Association. She is also a social psychologist and
serves on the Steering Committee of the Royal
Society of Medicine's forum for maternity and the
newborn. During the past 20 years of specialization, she has produced over 40 publications
on intrapsychic and interpersonal aspects
of reproductivity and her textbook *Psychological
Processes of Childbearing* (Chapman & Hall, 1991)
is in its fourth reprint. She teaches a variety of
professional training programmes and lectures
worldwide.

PREGNANCY THE INSIDE STORY

Joan Raphael-Leff

JASON ARONSON INC.
Northvale, New Jersey
London

THE MASTER WORK SERIES

1995 softcover edition

Library of Congress Cataloging-in-Publication Data: *pending*

ISBN: 1-56821-579-7

Manufactured in the United States of America. Jason Aronson Inc. offers books and cassettes. For information and catalog write to Jason Aronson Inc., 230 Livingston Street, Northvale, New Jersey 07647.

This book is dedicated to my mother, with love

Also to the memory of my father
and to my partner, sons and daughter
and others who have a place in my inner world

My thanks to all those who have shared with me
the inside stories of their pregnant desires or pregnancies.

Wheels within wheels, wombs within wombs,
Oscillating, figure/ground as perspective turns:
Mother-daughter-me — cord-links on a chain.
Each uniquely storied
Nestling Russian-doll
    dowried
Sorrow-sweet fruition cursed with Eden-pain.

Clocking lunar cyles of bloodshed or gestation
Ova ripen, surge and burst
In firstfruit tithe.
Narrowing womb-cone of past generation
Awaits procreation beyond our grasp. We three
Glistening seeds of Eve's sun-honeyed fig —
Eternal fractals on the female tree.

Contents

| Introduction

Once upon a time there was . . . a twinkle in an inner eye.

This is the story of pregnancy. Unlike most stories, this one begins at the very beginning or even before, with the psychic idea of conception and its destiny in a person's internal reality and external realization. This perspective differs from most psychoanalytic descriptions which take as their starting point the *infant's* developing psychological self. My central focus is on the *parent's experience* – the mother or father as a whole person rather than the object of the child's fantasy or desire. In the literature, granted little subjectivity of her own, a mother is often described in relation to the baby's needs. Yet if, as I believe, the very fabric of our early days is fashioned through interwoven subjectivities – carer's as well as infant's, unconscious as well as conscious – we cannot afford to leave out one part of the equation. Therefore, in this book, most of the time, the usual figure and ground will be reversed. Narratives of pregnancy and early infancy by mothers and fathers expressed from their own viewpoint will take the place of either the hypothetical baby's voice or that of the prescribing expert. Nevertheless, the story is never linear: we parents are also always sons and daughters in our own right. I therefore at times alter my focus to examine a fractal-like series of levels – from the internal world of the individual; to current interpersonal interaction with partner and/or baby, and as children to their own parents; moving beyond that to the realm of patient-therapist, and the relation of psychoanalytic theory to parenting.

There is irony in exploring the emotional processes of child bearing at this point in time, when the facts of life are changing more rapidly than our unconscious capacity to keep abreast of them. It is telling that so much attention has been paid to the biological aspects of reproduction, and so little to the rich seams of imagery, anxiety, and personal growth that accompany pregnancy. In this book I redress the imbalance by focusing on the 'inside' story.

Nor do all stories end 'happily ever after'. Inevitably, we shall venture into those areas where a conspiracy of silence has sustained fairy tales of blissful pregnancies, painless childbirth, perfect babies, and unconditionally loving parents. Here, as elsewhere, I have let people speak for themselves. Unless otherwise specified the quoted material is from psychotherapeutic records and verbatim notes from discussion groups and workshops. A few are transcribed from audio or video tapes. To maintain confidentiality I've chosen new names – a complex process akin to baby-naming – and disguised revealing details. Where applicable, permission has been obtained.

Supplementing thousands of hours of firsthand data are baby observations and clinical discussions with students I have taught, psychoanalytic psychotherapists I have supervised and, above all, the written work of mentors and exchanges with colleagues. As an informal backdrop, I am also informed by the experience of my own pregnancies, some of which occurred while in analysis myself, and of childbearing in a large number of ordinary parents whom I have come to know in a variety of situations of discussion, observation, group exploration, in-depth research interviews, or workshops and teaching.

Of all human practices, childbearing most emphasizes our basic gender differences, our common biological denominators worldwide and our cultural diversities. I am well aware of the limitations of an ethnocentric view. This book has been written while travelling over five continents between lectures and workshops for childbearing women and men, and health care professionals. As such, it has been influenced by my exposure to a variety of traditional and changing societal practices relating to pregnancy and childbirth.

Childbearing practices reveal a society's basic values and beliefs, as well as attitudes towards bodies, babies, women, and paternal roles. In each society, values are reflected in allocation of resources and the wide array of childbirth choices available – from wholesome home-births to underwater deliveries in darkened rooms to the sound of whistling dolphins, to state-funded projects that offer mother, father, and siblings a three-day 'baby moon' in a five-star hospital-hotel, to modernized, centralized, antiseptic births where compartmentalized women labour silently alone, without family members or even a midwife.

My *clinical sources* include close to two hundred pregnant women, expectant partners, and parents, seen individually or in couples in one- to five-times-per-week analysis or psychoanalytic psychotherapy for two to seven years each, or in on-going weekly therapeutic groups during pregnancy and the first year of motherhood. The *non-patient sample* includes many all-female or mixed groups, both lay and professional, seen in the context of workshops and discussion groups (many tape-recorded), which I have conducted here and abroad over the past eighteen years. In addition, for eight years I spent three mornings a week in a large parent-run playgroup I set up in 1977 within a London community centre, comprising some two hundred families. In this setting I participated daily in informal parental nattering, conducted systematic observation of twenty-three mother/baby pairs from infancy for two years, and three modest questionnaire studies at one-and-a-half year intervals (n=81), as the population changed.

Although this sampling is inevitably flawed by a middle-class self-selective bias, it does have an advantage in representing people who are economically freer to act from internal choice or compulsion rather than external necessity. Inevitably, a further bias is that of the dominant culture and colour. Nevertheless – unspecified for reasons of confidentiality – some of the individuals I quote are of Afro-Caribbean, Indian, or South American origin, in addition to others who have come here from various European or North American countries. Where appropriate, I focus on religious back-grounds or ethnic minorities in our own society, or illustrate a point with fragments from other cultures which question tacitly held theoretical presumptions of universality. It is pleasing that in recent years several larger-scale or longitudinal studies in the UK and in various countries abroad, – such as Israel, United States, China, Sweden, Japan, South Africa, Canada, and Hong Kong – are in the process of testing the models I put forth in this book, and I await their further findings.

Methodological flaws notwithstanding, above all I have endeav-oured to use my studies as a means of exploring parenthood and eliciting information rather than imposing value judgements or preconceived ideas. People differ: there are as many parenting styles as there are parents, and I have tried to express this diversity while also tracing similarities. The questions I have asked relate to psychosocial experiences and emotional processes of childbearing:

What meaning does childbearing have in the internal work of a woman or man? How do unconscious forces influence our becoming parents? What does it feel like to have another person inside you? What is an expectant partner's emotional experience of pregnancy? What do we know about fetal capacities and who/what does the fetus seem to represent for each parent? What are the emotions and dreams of pregnancy and which fantasies and fears surround birth? How do we become who we are in relation to our babies and our own baby selves? Do expectations of an imaginary baby dovetail with the one who arrives? How are we affected by exposure to the naked needs of a newborn? What happens to an intimate relationship when partners procreate? How does antenatal imagery affect the interactional climate postnatally? . . .

We shall explore the issues distilled in the questions above more or less in the order in which they appear here. The initial chapters discuss the emotional upheaval in internal worlds reflected in the fantasies and dreams of pregnancy. Then two related models are presented. The first – the placental paradigm – relating to the affect-laden connection of the pregnant dyad appears in Chapter 3. Following an examination of the place of paternity in Chapter 4, the model is fleshed out in Chapter 5 in terms of different unconscious configurations of the baby, and the effect of these on the experience of pregnancy. Chapter 6 describes a variety of changes in close relationships and attitudes to work during pregnancy and early parenthood. Chapter 7 focuses on how technological advances intercept the growing baby – real, imagined, threatened and sadly damaged or lost. Chapter 8 explores some of the fears, fantasies, and facts surrounding birth. Chapter 9 discusses different approaches to parenting and how these affect parenting beliefs and behaviour, seen once again through the Facilitator-Regulator-Reciprocator Model, introduced in Chapter 5 regarding pregnancy. Finally, in the penultimate chapter we look at pre- and perinatal psychotherapy and end in Chapter 11 by examining issues relating to psychotherapy in early parenthood. For therapists, an Appendix identifies people who may be at risk during the period of childbearing.

This whole area of procreation is highly charged, and human emotions are rarely simple. I have tried to convey some of the complex richness of mixed feelings and the variety of unconscious determinants that underpin our interactions. Clearly, given the individualized nature of our internal worlds, there can be no one 'inside story'. Although descriptive, my models try to capture the diversity of parental beliefs and behaviour, homing in on the plurality of motivational forces and symbolic processes in each individual while identifying certain clusters of meaning that are fairly consistent over time and across people who share the same parental 'orientation'. I have also allowed for dynamic shifts attributable to changes within the parent's internal world and psychosocial reality. Of necessity, at times for the sake of clarity, I have had to oversimplify or highlight certain features at the expense of others, to make a point. However, I have endeavoured to preserve some of the multilayered complexity of the many versions of our internal narratives.

In recent times we have come to realize that the female half of the human race has long been described in borrowed terms, and defined by concepts which have proved inappropriate. In a world of changing opportunities, mothers can no longer afford to be treated as selfless vehicles for nurturing and gratification of their offspring as advocated in the past, nor should they agree to be scapegoated as the cause of all their children's present and future difficulties. If we are to grasp our own experience, I believe we women can no longer be framed within a masculine model but must respond to the growing urge to take ourselves seriously – by listening to our inner voices, and speaking out our own truths and desires grounded in our unique 'psycho-bio-social' vicissitudes. Although translated into shared language, the meaningful significance of our subjective self-definitions can only evolve by contemplating the way we have internalized external values imposed upon us, and the ways in which having an actively reproductive female body shapes imagery and psycho-bio-social configurations in a woman's inner world.

Note that I say 'a woman' rather than 'women'; there is a tendency to treat mothers as though they constitute a common unified identity. I have attempted to illustrate some differences between expectant mothers, and the way in which each woman's female sex also intersects with familial, subcultural, ethnic, and local parameters to form her unique identity. Psychoanalysis itself began with accounts of female voices and 'speaking' bodies, yet in time those early patients of Freud's came to be replaced by male patients and standards. Given the predominance of men's voices in literature and social institutions, I make no apologies for the preponderance of female speech quoted in these pages.

If I have to highlight one conclusion from my work, it is that there can be no one premeditated Right Way. Each individual parent's and professional's orientation towards care giving reflects the current chapter of their cumulative inside story constantly written and rewritten in joint authorship with their intimates. To paraphrase Kermit the Frog, accepting that we are each the sum total of our life's stories, we can only take what we have and fly with it. In that spirit I offer this book.

1
Conceived Fantasies

A group of pregnant women relate their stories at a workshop:

'I was utterly convinced I was sterile when I didn't conceive the first time', says Rita, a teacher, early on in her pregnancy. 'Then I missed a period, but I still couldn't believe it, so I had an extra test to make absolutely sure.'

'Mine was an unplanned pregnancy', Nina says, stroking her twenty-three week 'bump'. 'It took me a while to come to terms with it, and even now I'm terrified I may have made the wrong decision.'

'When I had my coil removed, I imagined I wanted a daughter, thinking I'd dealt with all those old mother/ daughter tensions. But as soon as I became pregnant, every- thing was thrown up again. Now I dread having a girl', volun- teers Pat reflectively.

'Whatever my baby's sex, I believe its personality was for- ged by the passionate way it was conceived: in the white-heat longing, when David and I finally came together', Diana, who lives separately from her partner, tells the group.

'We were much more prosaic', replies Nancy, stretching her bare legs. 'As we turned thirty-five, I felt we were getting a bit long in the tooth, and said, "How about it?" Luckily, he felt the same, and my body responded despite my age.'

'You've all had it easy', says Andrea, who lives with her female partner. 'When we decided we wanted a baby, I had a terrible job finding a suitable donor for self-insemination. We didn't want frozen sperm, it's so impersonal . . . As it turned out, it was worth waiting – we found a super guy, who has become a friend, and, hopefully, will be attentive without being too intrusive.'

The Inside Story

A woman discovers she is pregnant. Having taken root in the

uterine space the miniscule, fertilized ovum will have a far-reaching influence in drawing the woman into the depths of her psychic space, tap-rooting powerful unconscious representations from her inside story which begin to permeate her dreams, fantasies and emotional life.

Conception is the beginning of a bizarre story. In pregnancy, there are two bodies, one inside the other. Two people live under one skin – a strange union that recalls gestation of the pregnant woman herself in the uterus of her own mother many years earlier. When so much of life is dedicated to maintaining our integrity as distinct beings, this bodily tandem is an uncanny fact. Two-in-one-body also constitutes a biological enigma, as for reasons we do not quite understand, the mother-to-be's body suppresses her immunological defences to allow the partly foreign body to reside within her. I suggest that psychologically too, in order for a woman to make the pregnancy her own, she has to overcome threats posed by conception. Its meaning flows from the placenta of her emotional reality embedded in the circumstances of her social reality.

The inside story differs for each pregnancy; every mother infuses it with her personal feelings, hopes, memories, and powerful unconscious mythologies. An imaginary baby is juxtaposed on the embryo implanting in her fertile womb. Even before conception, the unknown baby is drawn into an expectant woman's psychic reality, invested with illusion and ascribed a place among the many images of significant primary figures in her internal world. Under conditions of mental health, such configurations are rarely fixed: like the coloured bits in a kaleidoscope, constituents of the inside story are constantly being reactivated and processed, creating new formulations. In the turbulence of pregnancy, the continuous stream of internal narratives is simultaneously refracted through inextricably welded prisms of the psychic, physiological and social domains.

Each of us contains an inner world, inhabited by fluctuating fantasies and unconscious imagery from many versions of our internal relationships. Internal 'voices' may clash, and our various potentialities sometimes seem to engage in complex interaction among themselves. These highly personalized configurations not only colour our moods and perceptions, but at times inner conflicts and scripts come to be played out externally. People outside are enlisted to recreate emotional climates from the past by unconsciously acting in scenes we unconsciously allocate them. We each also unwittingly play roles in the expectations of others. Old themes are repeated as we unknowingly attempt to perpetuate and replay in external reality interpersonal exchanges which have not been resolved – trying to understand or make ourselves understood, or hoping to recapture a previous sense of self.

Thus, there is a continuous interweaving of external and internal realities, as through displacement, projection or the enactment of unconscious fantasies in the outside world, we actualize wishes and rid ourselves of intolerable states of mind. We make use of recurrernt patterns to get others to provide recognition, confirm our beliefs, materialize our apparitions, and feel our feelings or carry our burdens. Transformed, externalized aspects of ourselves are then taken back inside us to modify internal voices and representations, for better or for worse. Even when we are alone, mental life has a lively interpersonal substantiality despite its 'imaginary' quality, and some internal presences can be more real and influential than their flesh and blood counterparts. Lacking insight, we perpetuate old structures in new conditions, unable to break free of the grip of the past.

From the pregnant woman's point of view, another being has in actuality come to reside inside her as her body becomes physically occupied by another. The embryo is separate yet part of the woman's interior, already gendered, but to her of unspecified sex.

As Donald Winnicott says of the child's teddy or security blanket, we may say that the fetus belongs to that unchallenged, intensely imaginative intermediate area of experiencing to which inner reality and external life both contribute. Perhaps we may even go so far as to say of the fetus, as Winnicott states of the transitional object, 'that it is a matter of agreement between us . . . that we will never ask the question "Did you conceive of this or was it presented to you from without?" ' (Winnicott, 1951, p. 239). It is only as birth approaches that the inside story recedes. For example, twenty-three-year-old Rachel referred herself for therapy during pregnancy because of great anxiety. She felt she had to maintain continuous vigilance to keep the fetus alive, never for a moment allowing her thoughts to stray from it. This constant pressure is intensified by experiences of competitive rivalry with her mother and sisters whenever they meet, which she fears creates a hostile environment that endangers her baby.

However, even when she is alone Rachel has to ward off attacks from an image of her mother residing inside her, who is felt to be envious and resentful. She has spent her entire pregnancy convinced her baby is male and relating to him as 'the strong, special, brave little son' her father craved but never had. After months of therapy, it is now a few days before she gives birth (to a daughter):

> 'Labour is throwing something away. Why did I say that? No, labour is expulsion. No! It's like snakes shedding a skin. The baby inside is not the one that will emerge. The one I'll get is the real one, the inside one is fantasy . . . I'll miss him when he's born . . . Can something exist that can't be tangible or seen? . . . I look in the mirror and don't know who I'm looking at. The baby takes so much. Having another person in there leaves little room for myself, as if I can't be self-appraising while pregnant because I'm too absorbed in giving and listening in to the baby; my inner relationship with the baby . . . I am its medium . . . I'm afraid of not relating to the new baby after knowing this raw, slimy, throbbing baby inside.'

Rachel realizes that her fantasy baby will have to be relinquished if she is to greet the newborn one as a new individual. Nevertheless, we all to some degree continue to invest people in the external world with properties derived from our multiform internal figures. As we have seen, discrepancies between subjective psychic realities and shared social realities stem from the way in which we unconsciously select and transpose personal meanings between inner and outer worlds, resulting for each of us in individualized vision. Throughout our lives, these dynamics continue to fluctuate, change, regress, and mature as crucial images become assimilated, integrated into our identities, or remain unmetabolized foreign presences stuck inside or rejected, while others undergo repression or fade out of affective prominence in our interpersonal interactions.

When adults come together to form an intimate relationship, each person releases into it unresolved issues from their transgenerational pool of unconscious fantasies. Partners are often chosen to actualize certain potentialities for each other, and the unborn baby becomes party to their drama. Unrelinquished attributions will be incorporated by the newborn baby as part of his or her self-image, as the parents' preconscious configurations form the basis of the infant's internal world.

The baby's arrival arouses evocative memory fragments, revitalizing dormant processes related to the parents' own infancies, which influence the quality of postnatal interaction, as much as do their caring efforts. Conversely, the infant too propells his or her intense emotions into the care givers, unconsciously locking into existing structures in their internal worlds.

Even in the womb, exchange across boundaries occurs. Improved ultrasound visualization and fibreoptic filming has allowed us to observe the live fetus within the womb, actively ingesting and expelling, chewing, licking, and sucking body parts or the cord, yawning, pushing, kicking, and urinating. What is more, discrimination occurs: the rate of swallowing has been found to escalate dramatically when amniotic fluid is sweetened and is reduced when a bitter substance is injected into the fluid.

This absorption and regurgitation, taking in and spitting out has been regarded as a precursor to the way in which, once born, a baby gradually builds a sense of having an inside and an outside. But it seems to me that a baby does not arrive with preconceptions; understanding of the world and self-knowledge arise out of interpersonal exchange. The care givers are the life blood, and the environment the amniotic fluid. Through these the infant creates meaning, and their images gradually come to supplement actual relationships, impelled by fear of their loss or corruption. By identifying with beloved figures the baby can hold them inside the self for safekeeping, or they may also be internalized as a means of coping with or compensating for deficiencies of the real care giver. Thus, psychic realities of mother, father, and infant intersect and intermesh from conception and even before, contributing to the formation of a family culture.

Internal Conceptions

Conception may surprise a woman who finds herself pregnant when she has hardly begun to think about having a baby, or had time to recover from the last one, or had even been determined to avoid pregnancy. It may be the fulfilment of a long-held childhood dream, or reversal of her child-free existence. Pregnancy may fill an aching, inner void or reflect a broody baby hunger, or it may constitute an unwanted invasion. It may be a first pregnancy; a second or third to extend a family; a first with a new partner; or one replacing a previous miscarriage or loss. Conception may be motivated by a compelling need to undo the past, or change the future:

> 'I've had this strange desire to get pregnant again', says Rimona, when her baby is six months old. 'It's as though I'm needing to repeat something from the beginning, to get the essence of it – get it just right this time. With my first baby I was so depressed I missed out on her babyhood. With this baby, I've felt so involved, and so sad not to have been there fully with the first. Having a third would be striking out into the unknown – my mother only had two. I've also come from a mother who treats babies competitively: hers should be bigger and more advanced. I feel upset that I had to learn to be soft and loving and appreciative so late, that I had to learn it through other people rather than being instilled with it from having experienced it myself. If I did it again I'd have it in me from the start of pregnancy – that catch-in-the-throat "ah-h-h" people get when looking at a tiny baby . . .'

The pregnant woman may have no steady partner, or a relationship with a male lover, or one with a woman. Planned or unexpected, conception can delight both partners, only one, or neither – or occur in the context of a couple who do not equally welcome a child.

Unconsciously, pregnancy might represent the blissful fantasy of returning to symbiotic fusion in the womb; undoing primal dividedness; or providing proof of sexual desirability. Pregnancy may have little to do with the baby to come:

> 'I wanted to be pregnant so much that for all the long months I was trying to conceive I was so envious I couldn't look at a pregnant woman in the street', says Suzy, looking back. 'The state of being pregnant was my absolute aim in life. I couldn't look beyond the big bump. When I did conceive, I was over the moon! I can do it! I wanted to be pregnant, and didn't relate it to having a child – that was a real shock.'

The meaning of conception varies greatly, in different women and in the same woman over time. For Suzy, whose deprived childhood had left her feeling emotionally barren, exploited, and invisible, the state of pregnancy confirmed her creativity, filling her with wonder at her growing substantiality and presence. Longstanding emotional hunger and yearning to be recognized seemed finally satiated, and she revelled in the solicitous care and attention showered on her during pregnancy. Following the birth, however, she became severely depressed, feeling once again emptied and exploited, as her needy, demanding baby claimed a right to her resources for himself.

Timing is crucial. First conception may offer an older woman the cherished last chance to become a mother: 'With menopause looming, this pregnancy seems a doubly precious, unexpected gift', or might pose the life-upheaval threat of turning a teenage girl into one: 'My mother doesn't believe I could look after a baby myself, but I'm desperate to keep it.' It may come too late in a faltering relationship, too soon in a budding one. A woman on her own may have gone about seeking pregnancy methodically, carefully choosing a genetic father for her baby. Her urgency may have been due to a sense of emotional readiness or emptiness, midlife crisis, or a race against tyranny of the ovulatory sell-by date, an attempt to beat a deteriorating physical condition such as diabetes, pending hysterectomy, or HIV infection. Under such circumstances, having a baby may seem too important to postpone until she finds the right partner, and too precious to forgo in the absence of perfect conditions.

Depending on their closeness, and whom he represents in her mind, she may wish to share her news with the baby's biological father, or keep it to herself. She may have found herself pregnant or made a conscious choice to have a child, conceived through sex, professional intervention, or by self-insemination with donor sperm. She may even be serving as a surrogate womb. Some pregnancies follow rape or a casual relationship and involve agonized decisions whether to keep the baby, have an abortion, or give it away for adoption. In her eagerness to erase the father, a woman may deny his existence. In her fantasies, the pregnancy may be hers alone, rather than a coming together echoing the original parental couple who made her.

Undermining the rational control offered by thought and contraception, conception expresses an unconscious story of the body, reflecting lifelong ideas of child-bearing and representations of her procreative, female self. When a little girl has grown up in loving identification with a satisfied mother who takes pride in her own fertile, sexual body, and who has a pleasurable relationship with a partner she will feel permitted to have a child to express the fullness of her own life. This delicate balance between loving closeness and recognition of distinctness, however, is not always achieved. A dissatisfied mother might have used her daughter to plug the emotional emptiness of her own life, preventing acquisition of a *body image* that is distinctly unique. A hostile or envious mother may have prevented or interfered with the growing girl's enjoyment of her early feminine *sexual identity*, and both parents often fail to respond supportively to their adolescent's attempts to own their bodies. Once grown up, a daughter may feel compelled to use her body to play out internal preoccupations. She may, for example, belatedly try to break out of the maternal magic circle, yet seek a similarly intense emotional mutuality through a baby of her own: 'Its little hands will hold round my neck all the time, so close there's no need for words.' Or she may feel driven to forge separateness from mother through psychosomatic, nutritional, sexual, self-destructive, or reproductive bodily enactments which establish her autonomy. Here, Lucy illustrates how, by-passing thought, the female sexual body may be employed to enact internal conflicts:

> 'She never knew about my abortions, but I realize now they were directed at her', Lucy, an ex-photographer's model says sadly, with painful insight gained from hard work in psychotherapy some years after her mother's death. 'I never was real to my mother. She loved me more than anything in the world and told me everything, but I was her dolly, with no life of my own. Looking back, I'm so ashamed of my promiscuity, but it was the only way I knew to break free.'

Mysteries of Gestation

However conception occurs, and whatever the fate of the baby postnatally, pregnancy is a quintessentially female experience. Physically, it is in a woman's internal space that the baby is implanted; it is her body that will change. Psychically, the baby is implanted in the soil of her unconscious inner world, gaining substance from her fantasies, influenced by and influencing the climate of her psychic reality.

Who the woman is, and how, when, why, and with whom a baby is conceived sets the scene for reception of the pregnancy. Nevertheless, even the most joyfully anticipated conception entails some ambivalence, since creation of a new life also signifies loss of the old. As it becomes clear that her symptoms are not premenstrual but those of a budding pregnancy, even when much awaited, a woman may find her excitement tempered with trepidation about being swept along by the inexorable course she has taken. Suspending her reactions, in a determined effort to hibernate for fear something will go wrong, she may blankly refuse to engage emotionally with an unwanted pregnancy. These are extreme reactions. In general, the hallmark of pregnancy is a celebration of female resilience: those countless women throughout the ages who, alone in the dead of the night, have engaged with the emotional risk of trusting their own bodies to a process of growth over which they have so little control, whether in trepidation, or in affirmation of their faith that internal creative forces will prevail.

Reappraising Body and Self

While gestating her baby, a woman's freedom of choice is curtailed. For the duration of the pregnancy she must share her body with another who is always there, even in her most private moments; who interrupts her thoughts and disturbs her sleep, forces her to change her eating, working and toilet habits, and alters activity patterns of a lifetime. Women who have had a baby may be surprised by new anxieties and fears not experienced in previous pregnancies. When pregnancy is idealized and/or its affective aspects known only to initiated women, the degree of emotional upheaval and physical tiredness in early pregnancy may take a first-timer by surprise: 'I've never been so exhausted before – it's overpowering in a way I hadn't expected', says a doctor in her third month of pregnancy. 'When I mention it to other women, it's like entering a club, with everyone talking about their own experiences in pregnancy.'

Although the pregnant woman may welcome her rapidly changing shape, loss of her figure and familiar bodily responses means she can no longer anticipate her physical states nor can she control her appearance. Women who have suffered from eating disorders may have particular difficulty adjusting to a new body image. In addition to its size, her pregnant body discloses her secret life to all, proclaiming she is sexually active and fertile. In turn, strangers may feel entitled to pass remarks, or hand out unsolicited advice.

Pregnancy dissolves familiar connections between the woman and her body which have hitherto been taken for granted. She is no longer in sole possession of her own body. Its familiarity is altered in subtle and major ways. In her mirror, a fat, blue-veined interloper examines herself, watching and being watched by a stranger who looks out through her own eyes. Body sensations, too, feel foreign. An altered centre of gravity jerks her into floundering movements which defy control, impairing the sense of self in space. Pregnancy queers her balance, width-gauge, and aim. As bending in the middle becomes difficult, and her shambling feet invisible, gateways and parking spaces contract or expand erratically. Impressions are skewed by her sensory hypersensitivity. Her body odour changes; she smells different to herself. Indeed, her heightened sense of smell and close bodily receptors at times take precedence over distant cues. Temperature control, equilibrium, kinesthesia, complexion, hair texture, taste-buds, vision acuity, touch-pads, and extremities undergo unpredictable transformations, following some mysterious blueprint.

As pregnancy imposes constant revision of both sensory patterning and process representations, she has to reformulate her most elementary sensory experience, often having to reinvent old-new descriptive categories to capture these. Primitive concepts of bodily sensation revitalized during pregnancy hark back to the woman's own infantile experience. Reactivated and new excitations abound as she encompasses the unfamiliar shape, texture, and response of her estranged body, the bizarre sense of containing new organs and inner cavities, and the uncanny experience of another inside.

Continuity of self is disrupted by internal distractions which disturb her ordinary illusion of unified identity and indivisibility. Pregnancy throws into question body boundaries which since babyhood have defined the separateness of her own self within her own skin. Not only are her inner experiences now altered by heightened metabolic processes, but these are also punctuated by unpredictable activity and a diurnal rhythm not of her making. She is literally possessed by another: she throbs with the other's heartbeat, excretes his/her waste, is jolted into fitful waking, and stung to the quick with each lively quiver of the baby's being.

Day and night there is no respite. In fact, fetal movements seem to be strongest at the very times she is quiet, suggesting a cycle of interaction. She is acutely aware of this dual periodicity within her, intrigued by the baby's interconnected yet independent existence. Craving the time when she will be herself, she wonders whether she can ever again feel as unself-consciously singular as she did. Integrity takes on a different meaning now that she has become divisible.

Pregnancy exposes the woman to a primitive form of experiencing in which the known landmarks of ordinary bodily sensations and emotional organization shift and alter, at times falling into a formlessness with no fixed framework but the idea of her due date.

Transformational Phases

Although each pregnancy differs, I suggest we may distinguish three phases, each triggered by a transition, which may either further psychic change, or establish defensive coping mechanisms.

During the first phase of pregnancy, the woman is largely preoccupied with registering and adapting to new bodily sensations, symptoms, and emotional disequilibrium, and adjusting to the practical implications of her altered state. The second or mid-pregnancy phase begins with internal movements, when the emphasis shifts from the 'pregnancy' to the extraordinary idea of a separate and unknown being growing inside her. The third and final phase is initiated when the expectant mother begins to consider her baby to be viable, and could survive outside her if it was to be born prematurely. Thus, over the three trimesters, *the focus shifts from pregnancy, to fetus, to baby.*

Early Pregnancy

Even before conception, a woman who is sensitively in touch with her body may read the signs of her fertility: 'With my last baby, we had to keep making love the whole week for months', says Daniel's mother. 'This time, I distinctly felt a "ping" as I ovulated, and said to my husband, "We've got to do it tonight".'

During the first phase after fertilization, rapid cellular proliferation occurs with increasing differentiation and embryonic

organs begin to develop. At this time, early hormonal and metabolic changes produce minor symptoms, which the woman may
register even before knowing she has conceived, or recalls once
her period is late.

A woman may become aware of slight changes in the tenderness of her breasts, consistency of vaginal excretions, or the taste
of her saliva, described by some as metallic. She might experience
a slight tingling in her palms or soles, increased sweating, tiredness, breathlessness, or subtle alterations in the look and feel of
her skin and hair, and acuity of her sense of smell. On the other
hand, she may only have the impression of something that signifies pregnancy. Early awareness and increased confidence in
recognizing her subtle bodily signs can enhance the woman's
trust in her body's capacity to grow the baby, and to know how
to give birth:

> 'I can't define it,' says the doctor we encountered earlier, 'but I
> had an absolutely burning conviction I was pregnant, and al-
> though when I tested it there was only an ambiguous faint blue
> line, I persisted for days until, sure enough, it showed . . . I've
> always just taken for granted that my body gets me through the
> day, but hadn't appreciated how attuned to it I am.'

A newly pregnant woman often feels physically energized or
emotionally hyped up. Experiencing this excited wellbeing during the day, she may be surprised to find herself unusually fatigued and emotionally flat towards evening. Insomnia or early
waking may occur, as current activities are reappraised in the
light of changes to come, and her lifestyle changes to accommodate her symptoms:

> 'I do feel very different', says Hannah, a young professional in
> her seventh week of pregnancy. 'In the mornings I wake ear-
> lier and don't have that dread of daytime feeling of having to
> force myself out of bed like before. Even travel sickness is not
> too bad – in fact when I don't go in to work because of nausea,
> I think about what I'm missing at work rather than seeing it as
> a permanent life sentence because I'm not doing something
> better instead. And when I come back dead tired in the eve-
> nings, John is very kind. I just sit with my feet up while he
> cooks the supper.'

During the first phase of pregnancy, near-miss scares, or a history of previous miscarriages increases the sense of vulnerability. Many pregnant women feel they cannot relax until the watershed of the second trimester:

> 'I have a dilemma about telling my parents: my mother is unwell and low. Knowing I was finally pregnant again would chivvy her up and give them both an enormous boost, but then another miscarriage would be quite traumatic. There's such an irony that having been willing time to slow down while I tried to get pregnant, I'm now desperate for the next four weeks to pass so I can be sure', says Leah.

Mid-pregnancy

The hallmark of the second phase of pregnancy is an acknowledgement of the baby inside. During pregnancy, two people occupy one space. As this realization dawns, the pregnant woman must reverse all she has striven to establish since her childhood: despite dreams of emotional fusion, people are separate; each inhabits his or her own body, and each is either male or female. Not only is there another being inside her, but it has about a fifty-two per cent chance of being male. Even if female, it is comprised of a male contribution as well as her own.

Over the next months, the expectant mother has to tolerate sharing her body, while accepting that the lodger she bears is separate and beyond her control. Coming to terms with having two people under her skin is further complicated by a sense of triple identification: as the baby in her womb comes into focus, the woman cannot help but see the parallels with herself as a fetus in her own mother's womb. The current configuration of her emotional relationship to her archaic womb-mother will have unconscious bearing on the feelings she has about her own baby.

Symptoms such as nausea and fatigue diminish as the placenta becomes well established. Most mothers experience a great sense of physical wellbeing during the coming months, when, although the bulge becomes more noticeable, it is not yet uncomfortable. Although jolted out of deep sleep by severe nocturnal calf cramps (relievable by massage while stretching and flexing the toes) and a frequent need to urinate, her body is still her own.

Many women find themselves relaxing as they pass the thirteenth week, feeling the pregnancy is now secure:

> 'Before, I felt that if I moved too much the baby would drop out', says Ingrid in Sweden, echoing second-trimester feelings all over the world. 'Now that we've passed the three-month stage, and I don't feel sick, I can do whatever I like. It feels like being "me" again. Funny, I almost feel less pregnant than before.'

As movements from within increase, the woman often finds her attention divided between the demands of the external world and the bids for attention from within. She may invest the baby with characteristics, a pet name, likes and dislikes. Many women have silent conversations with the baby, or talk out loud to it, like an imaginary friend.

Continuing tenderness of her breasts reminds the woman of similar feelings she had in her pubescent body. In early adolescence, then as now her body image had to accommodate rapid physical changes, and become more womanly. Pregnancy constitutes a further stage in identification with the fertile, sexual, and now life-bearing body of the archaic mother. Paradoxically, at this time of creating a family of her own, accompanied by a thrust towards becoming a fully-fledged adult, she is also most aware of her vulnerable child self, the little girl she was, and still at times feels herself to be.

The pregnant woman who has had responsibilities prematurely thrust upon her in childhood may feel this is a last opportunity to let her little-girl self have a taste of carefree childhood before having to look after her own baby.

> 'My mother treats me as a big lazy lump if I put my feet up', Helena, a social worker, says sadly. 'Actually, I'd love to be looked after, but she wants me to care for her. All these years I've kept alive an illusion that one day she would recognize my needs, but I'm beginning to realize I can't change her. She's never going to be what I want her to. She's still engrossed in trying to make her own mother treat her differently, and seems to see me as a representative of her mother. She's always wanted to be fêted and pampered by me, and all I can do is set a limit on her demands and look after myself.'

Women who move happily back and forth between child and adult selves may feel at ease to lark about even while engaged in the grown-up activity of growing a baby. Previously inhibited women may experience pregnancy as liberating:

'I love the freedom of pregnancy', says Olivia, an accountant. 'Being so different from everyday life, it has no rules. I feel I can be anything I want. I put on funny voices, wear strange clothes, read books I wouldn't usually read, and indulge myself with luxurious bath oils, midnight feasts – saying or doing just anything that takes my fancy.'

If she comes from a family where pleasures were taken in secrecy, a woman who does not feel permitted to enjoy her feminine sexual identity may begin to feel alarmed as her expanding belly discloses her secret to the world. In situations where she is self-consciously aware of others observing her, feeling awkward and betrayed by her bulge, she may freeze up and find it difficult to rejoice openly. Where slimness and appearance have been central to a woman's self-image, it is not uncommon to find anxiety about losing her recognizable shape. She may have to make a conscious effort to adjust to the outward manifestations of her bodily changes, and remind herself of their cause.

As the fetus becomes more vigorous and clearly its own person, the woman comes to differentiate herself from the baby inside, and from her internal mother as well. This internal shift, which may not occur in first pregnancy, is accompanied for many women by a change in perspective which affects the external relationship to her mother, if she is alive. Paradoxically, acknowledgement of herself as joined to, yet separate from, the life growing inside her, and similar to, yet different from, the mother in whom she herself grew, can increase a woman's sense of responsibility for her own wellbeing, and therefore for that of the baby inside her. Tender care of her body deepens with increasing trust in her capacity to sustain, grow, and give birth to a healthy baby whom she can care for. Accordingly and conversely, awareness of her responsibility and ownership of her thoughts may lead to individuation:

'I've never known what I want', says Hannah, whom we met early in her pregnancy, now in the second trimester. 'I always find it so hard to make decisions. Being pregnant makes me have to think about things more honestly – I had a dream that my belly popped and the baby was lying there flattened, as if at the bottom of a shopping-bag. I woke crying and asked my partner to check if my belly was still round. I realize I dreamt it because I'm afraid I'll get worn out. I went dancing on the weekend and don't know if I should feel guilty because it was too much? I don't really know when I've had enough. I don't want to seem lazy and stop work too early, but I must leave myself enough time to relax. I don't know when I'm tired. In the early months when I was so exhausted, I just collapsed into bed because I couldn't do otherwise. Now I try to think what I've done in the day, and whether I've eaten properly, and if I should put my feet up and rest. I would find it so much easier if there was a list of what to do or not to do, but in its absence, things just happen. Except that now I'm responsible for someone else in there too, so I do have to take account and try and find out what I need.'

The Final Phase

'I feel frightened about the labour. I've got to get this baby out, but how will I feel about doing it? I'm scared. It's only three more months, but the baby might come early. I'm not ready, and want this stage to last longer. Right now I'm not too huge and tired. I feel very strong and rather placid. I like being pregnant. I'm happy with the way I look, and feel pleased and unself-conscious about my shape. But when the baby comes out, I'll feel flat and deflated and depleted. The way I am now I feel very self-contained and my mother's criticisms say nothing to me, but I'm afraid I might revert afterwards. I imagine her prodding my flab and snaping, "There's nothing there – get rid of that!" ', says Helena.

As the pregnant woman begins to consider that were her baby to be born prematurely, it would be viable, the end of pregnancy becomes a reality in her mind, and she enters the last phase. Bending in the middle becomes virtually impossible. Her belly is now heavy and large enough to get in the way while making love or driving. Only in the brief weightlessness of swimming or in dreams can the pregnant woman regain a sense of her old body.

The body space she shares with her baby has become cramped. Many women feel clumsy, full-blown and overworked, experiencing the need to slow down. Working mothers-to-be who can afford to do so often choose this point to go on maternity leave, making mental and practical space to relish the last baby-free period, and/or 'nesting' by preparing an external replacement-womb for the baby.

As the pregnancy progresses towards its end, the expectant mother usually becomes more aware of the momentous, irreversible change that is about to occur. The moment of truth looms large, with anxieties about the mutual journey they are about to take: 'This baby is really scrabbling about inside', says Rebecca at seven months. 'It's so active that I'm not sure it'll wait it out, but I'm scared and don't feel prepared at all.'

The last month or so are a mixture of cutting down on social demands, while escalating prebaby and preparatory activities, as anxiety mounts about completing all the arrangements before the birth. The baby's room and paraphernalia, odd house chores that can be put off no longer and tying up loose ends – like meeting all the community midwives in the team, reading the relevant books, or attending the last antenatal classes. Some expectant mothers frantically grab at cultural events, desperately aware of lifestyle changes to come. Commitments made so easily months before suddenly seem insurmountable, diverting her from the circle of her belly, and a parallel withdrawal into the enveloping circle of family and friends:

'My mind has turned to jelly. I've given it permission to slow down, and feel that it's a terrible effort to find words, and a monumental task to just concentrate', says Rebecca, now eight months pregnant. 'Last time I almost hadn't realized that pregnancy would end. I was like a ship in full sail, and enjoyed being the centre of attention. This time I want to withdraw. There's a greater feeling of reality about it – I'm excited and looking forward to knowing the baby, like unwrapping a present. Before my daughter was born, I had no idea about babies. The only ones I'd seen were on a hospital visit, and I thought of them as tiny, ugly, helpless, rubbery, disconnected things – I suppose like my little sister looked to me. It took me ages to feel differently about Lily when she was born. Now I can imagine the baby, but I'm still frightened about the birth:

how will I cope with two? Will the labour be difficult? Will we be ready for the baby?'

In the last few weeks, the pregnant woman often suffers from breathlessness, lassitude, constipation and heartburn. Her ligaments are stretching in preparation for the birth, and practice contractions, hardening her belly as she goes into spasm, become stronger and more frequent. As she waits, she is aware that the baby, too, is finishing its preparation for birth, priming systems needed for the transition to extra-uterine life, building up tissues and laying down fat deposits. The prudent mother-to-be may herself feel she is utilizing the remainder of her pregnancy to prepare for the birth, building the emotional resources and material provisions needed for transition to the demanding postnatal activities as the mother of a newborn baby living outside her.

> 'After the terrible labour I had last time, I feel a bit like an athlete – I need to eat well and rest well, limber up and prepare through training, to be in the best possible condition for what I know is hard work. And I've already laid on extra help for when I get home to help me through those excruciating first weeks', says Daniel's mother.

Faced with the unknown, and as the tension of uncertainty increases, most women indulge in superstitious monitoring of birth dates or days of the week. Like all magical ideas, these are an attempt to put some predictability into the unknown stretching ahead. Similarly, internal conflicts are projected into external happenings, with attendant moodiness, heightened emotions, and irrational fears of 'Divine retribution': 'I'm so afraid of my waters breaking, of being messy. There's a constant struggle with those voices telling me I'll never get away with it. I'm sure I'll flunk the birth test, or be the one who gets the monster', says Dora, who wants a caesarean.

Sometimes compulsion to retreat to the familiarity of the internal world overrides the threat of having to face the novelty of uncertainty. A woman may be so enmeshed in the emotional web of her family of origin that she is unable to make use of the generative base of pregnancy to assert her individuality. During delivery she may unconsciously repeat labour and birth patterns of women relatives, or of her own mother's parturition with a sibling in the equivalent birth order to this baby.

As she counts the days, eager anticipation may mingle with sorrow at losing the fantasy baby and specialness of pregnancy, with a foreboding of emptiness and fears of failure. Others, feeling ugly, exploited, and encumbered by the weight, cannot wait to get rid of the burden.

2
Pandora's Box

What of the end, Pandora? Was it thine
The deed that set these fiery pinions free? [. . .]
What of the end? these beat their wings at will,
The ill-born things, the good things turned ill—
Powers of the impassioned hours prohibited.
Aye, hug the cascet now! Whither they go
Thou may'st not dare to think: nor canst thou know
If Hope still pent there be alive or dead.

Dante Gabriel Rossetti, 'Pandora'

Hugging the 'casket' of her pregnant belly, a woman returns to her creative origins. Like Pandora's, the opening of an expectant mother's 'box' is associated with awakening of dormant passions and a release of internal ambivalence.

In Sorrow . . .

Sandra, a social worker, comes to see me in mid-pregnancy with severe depression. She says, 'I'm nobody and the baby seems more important than me – it has everything and I have nothing.' She expresses her fear of the envied baby becoming 'a monster', and, in the absence of friends and partner to centre her, anticipates herself acting out 'craziness' alone with the child for hours on end – an indefinable 'essence of witchness'.

Sandra feels her own 'harmonious' childhood went wrong when her adored father was often away on business. As an only child, during his absences she felt abandoned, left alone with her close-tongued, bustling mother who had 'standards to keep up', since her own house-proud mother was very self-sufficient, having been widowed during the First World War.

Gradually it emerges that Sandra is grieving for a previous lover who became independent and abruptly ended their exclusively intimate relationship. He left 'harbouring bitterness', although she had for years been a protective and all-providing bountiful 'mother'. On the rebound, she became pregnant soon after meeting her current partner. In the following months, as she uses the once-weekly therapy to talk through the 'forbidden' topic of her previous relationship, Sandra's copious tearfulness and insomnia lessen. She begins to see connections between him and her beloved father, who would not stay home despite all her devoted (manipulative) efforts.

The baby too is destined to leave her with birth. Gradually emotional investment in the baby within her swelling belly grows in inverse ratio to the diminishing preoccupation with abandonment. At first, although full of pregnancy, she feels empty, depleted, and furious with her impregnator. Despite valuing their healthy relationship, she scorned her 'down-to-earth' partner, who sees her clearly and realistically while she still yearns for the passionate excitement of that elusive relationship when she felt put on a pedestal and very special in spite of the anguished frustration and pain.

Craving the intense feelings she once experienced, she makes attempts to communicate with him, but her previous boyfriend is guarded, afraid she'll engulf him again and ask too much of him. Sandra remains obsessed with needing his recognition; his affirmation that the person she was still exists, and has not been wiped out in his mind. She is hurt that he regards her as a dangerous threat, but feels he is too fragile to be treated heavy-handedly. Following this failed contact, she no longer weeps but feels 'dry' – lonely, and choked, and unable to cry. She develops cystisis and feels poisoned by the invading fetus.

By thirty weeks the baby is much more active, has a pet name and definite personality, and as Sandra begins to acknowledge her need for rest, she tries to divert resources from her frantic busy-ness. She wakes from a disturbing dream in which her mother's mask-like face is reflected in the mirror Sandra herself is gazing into. She realizes that, like her mother and grandmother before her, she is in danger of becoming managing and stoic in the course of protecting herself from pining for an absent man, while neglecting the present.

After an enjoyable afternoon of gardening with her partner, it comes as a revelation to her that ordinary life can be good, and that the capacity to live it to the full instead of exciting peaks and dips of frustration and waste resides inside her rather than in external events. She finds the sensation of little limbs stirring within her strange and miraculous, saying she used to hate her bodily changes, and now can't imagine not being pregnant. As the baby's head becomes engaged in preparation for the birth, she tells me for the first time that with her previous lover she had had a very early miscarriage, following which he in effect had become her baby, as she possessively used him to compensate for her loss. Now, sobbing bitterly in the session for all her losses – absent father, preoccupied mother, jilting lover, unmourned baby – she releases this pregnancy from the grappling hooks of her past unfinished business. Sandra feels a great need for space – as if 'starved of the countryside' – and goes away for a few days with her husband on a long overdue honeymoon. Their little boy is born a few days later, two weeks early . . .

Permeability

In the early weeks after conception, a woman's attention may wander during the day, as semiconscious daydreams or anxious thoughts break through into consciousness. As psychoanalytic researchers such as Helene Deutsch, Grete Bibring, Judith Kestenberg and Dinora Pines have noted, while heightening awareness of bodily sensations, pregnancy churns up primitive anxieties and revitalizes emotions that had been laid to rest. For the woman who is able to take the risk and make use of the momentum, the very accessibility of hitherto repressed material offers a unique opportunity to explore her internal world.

In his *Psychopathology of Everyday Life*, Freud illustrated how seemingly bungled actions are actually successful compromise formations, allowing unconscious wishes and forbidden ideas to slip out, evading the internal censor. During pregnancy, slippages and oversights are often found to make symbolic sense, as do dreams and symptoms. Losing her purse or locking herself out might reflect the pregnant woman's ambivalent feelings about her 'inmate' taking over the inner 'purse' of her uterus, and using her resources while occupying her body. Pressurized by a society which glorifies pregnancy, denying her ambivalence, the woman may feel compelled to hide negative feelings – even from herself – to maintain the idealized, blissful state she is meant to experience. Some sleights of hand or faulty actions have a secondary gain in obstructing plans, expressing her resentment at having to be radiant while feeling depleted, or, conversely, to behave as usual despite the extraordinary change occurring within.

In ordinary daily life, we tend to filter out a great deal of stimuli, focusing on what appears to be most pertinent at the time, screening out irrelevant information from within and without. Mental and psychical pressure to re-examine her identity causes the pregnant woman to become more keenly aware of a wide range of sensations and subliminal impingements that she would normally exclude from awareness. Involuntary permeability of the boundaries between different levels of consciousness mean she is at times flooded with fantasies and ideas which previously were unconscious. She may feel unusually tearful, moody, or uncharacteristically emotional. Her temper may erupt in an unexpectedly volatile way, followed by tender remorse. She may be shocked to find that reawakened persecutory anxieties provoke superstitious or magical solutions.

Some women exert self-control and rigidify their internal barriers against this overdose of sensitivity, while others give in and enjoy the sensation of freewheeling. The loosening of defences and loss of emotional control may feel somewhat alarming. However, the disequilibrium of pregnancy has some spin-offs, often manifested in heightened sensuality and sensitivity to touch, smell, and colour, coupled with increased sensibility to the subtleties of emotional interaction, and a keener awareness of her own and other people's deepest feelings.

The Dream's Navel

Entering the dream world at night, we each partake of another existence in which the impossible becomes possible and the forbidden permissible. We play with imaginary versions of past and future realities, and allow ourselves glimpses of a rich and hidden world. Loosening the grip of rational cohesion, the dreamer self constructs new integrative patterns and permutations.

A dream serves to fulfil unconscious wishes while protecting sleep, as Freud suggested, with the internal censor making use of mechanisms such as displacement, condensation, and revision to transform and distort unconscious ideas and day residues into acceptable form. Dreams seem to serve a function of communicating with oneself, and by dramatizing internal representations – like a theatrical performance – can convey messages in a graphic and creative way. In our dreams, we tend to give symbolic expression to 'hot' anxieties and conflicts, which in their

disguised shapes can be unconsciously worked through and resolved. Persistent, unresolved anxieties may manifest in recurrent
dreams, or a series of dreams on similar themes. A further use of
dreams seems to be the working through and assimilation of
undigested experience, and its eventual integration into the
psyche. By allowing oneself to drift through various associations
to elements of the dream, further work may be done by the
dreamer upon waking, in reconstituting the original unconscious
content and translating it into conscious thought.

Dreams during pregnancy tend to be unusually plentiful,
vivid, and, at times, overwhelmingly realistic. They often persist
into waking life, leaving the dreamer feeling as if her internal
reality could take over the external one. Dreams reflect both
secrets of the primordial world of pregnancy, and longstanding
personal fantasies and anxieties about the sufficiency of her internal and external resources.

Freud and Jung suggested that some recurrent symbols
appear in myths, folklore legends and graphic art across the
generations and cultures, seeming to represent primal fantasies:
doors, gateways, and openings tend to represent body orifices,
such as the vagina; vessels, pots, cauldrons, and grails suggest
wombs; water often is associated with birth and/or sex; and
sleep with death.

In studying dreams reported by pregnant women in different
societies, it appears they share a common primal experience.
Although there are obvious methodological dangers in doing so,
it seems, distilled, myriad individual narratives can be seen to
express a few core experiences related to the fertile, shared, and
changing body; birth and mothering anxieties and maternal unpreparedness; intense love-hate relationships; and fear of death.

Despite psychosocial differences, many pregnant women may
be seen to be engaged with existential concerns about restricted
individual freedom and assymetry of needs following birth of the
dual-one into two. A sense of unpreparedness for the practical
implications of the imminent uncoupling of baby and self is
reflected in loss of the pregnant body as 'vehicle', which has been
taken for granted as the means of transporting and automatically
caring for the baby.

'My bicycle was taken. I think somebody stole it. I could not
go to work. I had to take the baby to my mother, but my

man's bicycle has no seat. My mother cannot come to me, and I cannot go to her', recounts Chu, in her third trimester, through an interpreter, in an antenatal clinic in China.

'I dreamed my baby had arrived', narrates Gabriella in her twenty-fourth week of pregnancy. 'It was small but very nice, and I wanted to go out but I hadn't yet bought a car seat. I couldn't leave the baby, but couldn't take it out, and I couldn't go myself to buy one. I woke in an incredible panic as there seemed absolutely no solution. Only a few days later did it occur to me I could have taken a bus.'

Like all others, dreams during pregnancy are intensely personal and reflect the dreamer's own idiosyncratic style of creative imagery and narrative peppered with residues of his of her experience of recent events and those of long ago. As such, each dream is a highly individual creation which can only be interpreted in the light of that particular dreamer's own associations to it. Nevertheless, in analysing dreams of pregnant women, I have traced a few basic themes which seem to recur in different cultures, although clearly the manifest symbolism varies according to the dreamer's local language of signs and metaphors, and her own individual fantasy style. I have clustered these in five overlapping categories.

Creativity and Elemental Opposites

The pregnant woman is engaged in an activity as old as human existence; it thrusts her into contact with the primal constituents of psychic life: female and male, birth and death, creativity and destruction, order and chaos, inside and outside. Although female she houses the male contribution and possibly a male fetus; although real and concrete she has little knowledge of her fetus; life-giving, she is potentially also death-dealing. She who was contained is now the container; she who was little is now big, and creating someone little. Her oneness is replaced with two, forcing a new kind of confrontation between self and other, fusion and separateness. All these are addressed in various story-lines and symbolic forms, such as giants and miniatures, barely disguised phallic symbols, vaginas and wombs, primitive landscapes and lush exotic jungles, creative beginnings burgeoning into life, or withering in saddening endings.

Feminine Mysteries and Birth

Pregnancy immerses a woman in the mysterious female processes of conception, gestation (formation, preservation, and
transformation), birth, and nurturing. Despite increased scientific understanding and incredible technological innovations, we
still grapple with generativity as a magical and enigmatic process.
Doubts about her capacity to contain, sustain, and keep the little
fetus which mysteriously must be transformed into a baby
mingle with rage at her absolute sense of aloneness.

> 'In my dream, the floor of my living-room was covered in
> strange marks on a black-and-red grid that I knew had super-
> natural significance, although I found them hard to decipher.
> Suddenly, an intruder got in and massacred my family, while I
> managed to escape through the back door, where a dwarf told
> me he'd been poisoned by listeria, and it was my fault.'

Like the birth to come and, ultimately, her own death, gestation is
a process in which no one else can participate. In her dreams she
may strive to share her solitary responsibility by dreaming her
partner or mother is pregnant for her; she may express anxieties
about the precariousness of her pregnancy by dreaming of her
belly deflating, internal bleeding, or menstruation. The fears about
the baby's viability or normality and her own capacity to nurture
may be reflected in dreams of losing the baby or forgetting to feed
him/her; preoccupation with deadlines and missing them, or tests
that are failed reflect an anxiety about being caught short, an
unreadiness for the birth and unpreparedness for the baby. During
the last trimester in particular anxiety dreams are more overtly
about the birth, for example, in images of the baby coming out of a
different orifice, getting stuck, vanishing or causing internal
damage. Here, a mid-European woman in her fifth month of
pregnancy recounts her dream of the previous night:

> 'I was in a twisty-turny corridor. It felt like going down but it
> was really up. It was like being in the tube tunnels at rush-
> hour, propelled along, swimming with the stream, yet trying
> to preserve my personal space. Then I got to the top of a
> helter-skelter. I stopped, unsure whether I should go down,
> afraid to give in and let go, in case I'd never be able to come
> back.'

As she brings her associations to the dream, it seems to express her identification with the baby struggling to be born, as well as her own mixed feelings about being midway in pregnancy and beginning to give up her professional life. In her last month of pregnancy, the same woman tells of another dream. No longer interchangeable, both she and the baby are part of the same process, inexorably moving towards the (b)end of pregnancy:

'I was riding a bike with the baby. I can't explain it, but it seemed I was 'one and a half'. As I approached a bend, I was going very fast and didn't know if I could make it. All I could do was hold on and hope for the best. I made it round, but my boyfriend was angry with me for taking a risk.'

Her associations are to having reached the turning-point of an emotional leave-taking, fast approaching the end of pregnancy. Looking forward to it, while also dreading being carried away by labour, she wonders how much she can trust her body, or even trust herself to not fight her body for fear of being 'thrown off balance' during the birth, or trying to do what others expect rather than what she feels. In the event, she had a relaxed water-birth, and produced a delightful baby.

Reappraisal of Identity

On a deep, unconscious level, the pregnant woman hovers between internal and external worlds, at a crossroads of past, present and future; self and other. The issue of a changing identity is crucial and disturbing, and often is expressed in Alice-in-Wonderland-type dreams of experiences of mutable, fluctuating shapes, sensations, and perception:

'I can't imagine a real baby being born, but I did have a dream about labour. Except instead of ordinary labour, horrible, fat, anaemic-looking tubular hairs grew out of the pores on my legs, oozing out like skinny penises, sort of bean-shooty things, squishy and almost translucent, but these were tree-like and branching . . . People think I'm calm, but I feel exposed and out of control, horrible hidden bits of me popping out. I'm murderous and vicious inside, and won't be able to hide from the baby', says a woman who is racked by internal doubts.

The Eternal Triangle

Pairs and triads, exclusion and inclusion, issues of rivalry, envy, jealousy, love and hate are played out in stark simplicity, or elaborately disguised scripts, as parents, siblings, and figures from the far past are juxtaposed with current and future events, enacting emotional intrigues:

> 'I've had awful vague nightmares in which my younger sister figured. There was a dark sense of danger, threatened violence, and a fire alarm with buttons for Police, Fire, Ambulance, Mother. I had to save myself from someone who was after me, but I couldn't get up or out.'

Fantasy Baby

Given the paucity of clues about the identity of her baby, the pregnant woman spins fantasies about the child in her womb who may appear in many human and animal guises. The primitive, involuntary nature of the birth process is often apparent, and, paradoxically, may symbolize delivery not of the baby, but of an internal child or the pregnant woman giving birth to a vital aspect of herself:

> 'Sometimes when I wake up I feel as if I've forgotten everything I thought I knew, as if it's all been wiped out, and then I start talking and realize I still can talk. Last night I dreamed I was swimming with dolphins, and had to let go of myself and dive down despite my fear of drowning. Then I got to an underground tunnel, and was wandering through dark, dank corridors. My mother came through a little door carrying a girl baby, although I am expecting a boy.'

Such dreams may pervade sleep with shadowy images, or zap her back into primal experiences. Some days she may feel so disorientated that she has the need to be surrounded by familiar things, to be cosy and safe at home. In many cases, dreams have the quality of a persistent message from within, some piece of emotional information conveyed in the face of resistances, or worked through with variations in successive dreams.

The Baby Real and Imagined

Unconscious fantasy is a constant accompaniment to our rational thoughts. It forms a mental grid or set by means of which we order our perceptions and structure our worlds. Even before birth, parents begin to ascribe characteristics to their baby, partly based on discernible fetal rhythms and responses and partly on fantasy. In the absence of clearcut evidence, the mother and father invest the 'bump' with an imaginary baby of their own making. Although they may not share each other's preference, many parents have a conscious wish for a dream-baby, with a particular appearance, personality, gender, and even name. Others are unaware of preferences, but know what they do not want. Although desires may become conscious, their origins lie in the swirling mists of the unconscious; the womb becomes a receptacle for hopes, wishes, desires, and anxieties as the baby is invested with properties of the parent's inner world.

The imaginary baby can represent a shadowy aspect of the parent's internal reality – a cherished or feared potentiality of themselves, or a vague image related to some significant figure from the past. A persecutory or damaging internal image may colour the experience of the fetus as a physical presence. A loving partner can mitigate some of these emotional difficulties. However, he or she too may have an internal world of persecutory figures who fill the pregnancy and early parenting with dark images of foreboding rather than optimism.

Early identifications and unresolved conflicts with the pregnant woman's archaic parents surface at this time of transition from being the child of her mother to being the mother of her own child. As she starts on the course of actualizing her wish for a baby, fantasies are reactivated relating to her early envy of her fertile mother, and jealousy of the parents' special relationship from which she was excluded. If she had younger siblings, impressions of her pregnant mother and memories relating to their birth are rekindled, as are old rivalries, and unconscious anxieties about maternal retaliation for daughter's desires, rage, and secret destructive wishes against the mother's babies.

As a result of these painful conflicts, the woman may have been left feeling guilty, ineffectual, and uncreative by comparison to her mother, inhibiting wanting a baby of her own for fear of having to pay too heavily. As in childhood, some pregnant women unconsciously make a secret pact, cautious about outdoing mother. Assuming she will not be allowed to keep everything without sacrificing something, she may feel compelled to relinquish sex, ambition or career in order to have the baby, or to hand her child over to her mother or substitute care giver.

Early misgivings arise in the context of unconscious pressures from significant others. The receptivity of powerful parents to a little girl's passionate early desires – and especially the meaning she herself attributed to their responses – will have coloured the sense of her own creative agency. The reaction of her partner, whom she may have unconsciously chosen to perpetuate parent-type transactions, or negate them, will affect her current belief in her life-engendering powers. In fact, the reverberations from the past, and figures who live on inside her inner world are often more influential than those she encounters in her daily life. Likewise, ingrained childhood evaluations, such as denigration of her creative capacities may override adult achievements and reality feedback, which in pregnancy can manifest in excessive anxiety, and a constant need for medical or emotional reassurance. During pregnancy she seeks confirmation that she is growing the baby correctly; that it is viable and normal, and has found a good place inside her and sufficient placental provisions.

Psyche and Soma

As the fetus is dependent on the quality of placental feeding in the womb, so for the pregnant woman internal images and unconscious historical factors constitute nutrients or toxins in her 'emotional placenta' conditioning mental gestation of her pregnancy.

For some, the intimate connection between psyche and soma may become so unbearable during pregnancy that a woman who cannot tolerate her own ambivalent feelings or the idea of sharing her body may have to resort to psychic expulsion – blanking out fantasies, and denying the baby a mental reality by refusing to acknowledge the child's coming into being. Or she may rid herself of the anticipation of becoming a mother, when this feels forbidden. Other women wrestle bodily with their internal conflicts:

'When I found out I was pregnant,' says Dora, a woman who referred herself for psychotherapy because of intolerable anxiety states during pregnancy, 'I was overjoyed at the miracle; then I began attacking myself mentally – I couldn't sleep and had the worst dreams and panic attacks and felt like cutting myself. I'm afraid I'm doing something wrong by wanting a baby – my mother hated having me, and thinks I should go ahead professionally and achieve what she was unable to. I fear harming the baby with my thoughts – I had some bleeding early on, and am convinced I'd caused it.'

Sometimes a pregnant woman's psychological reaction leads to the destruction of the embryo by elective abortion. Alongside the fetus, what is being aborted may be a disowned part of her internal world – which returns with a vengeance of guilt and self-recriminations. Anguished doubts and ambivalence may contribute to early miscarriage. Conflicts about an unplanned conception, symbolic equation of the embryo with something unwanted in herself, or a sense of having too few resources to sustain a child, may combine with physiological processes to end the pregnancy.

There is, however, no simple psychosomatic connection. Many unwanted pregnancies thrive despite internal opposition. Conversely, nausea and bleeding are not uncommon, even in the most wanted pregnancies. The important factor is how these and other physical symptoms are emotionally interpreted by the woman. A troubled woman may experience her sickness as an attempt to rid herself of the parasitic invader by being violently ill; another may feel she vomits because of being poisoned by the harmful fetus. An anxious woman may treat nausea as a sign of her internal insufficiency; a depressed one may feel it is her internal 'badness' being disgorged. Some women welcome ongoing symptoms as a definite indication that they are still pregnant. Constipation may unconsciously represent a fear of expulsion of the pregnancy, or a sense of static bunged-upness, or persecutory fantasies of merciless, internal demolition. This is not to say that symptoms are determined by feelings, but that the pregnant woman's response to them is affected by the symbolic meaning she unconsciously attributes to her physical state, which in turn may exacerbate symptoms or her anxious awareness of them.

Outside and Inside

Food is an intermediary between outside and inside, seeming to provide some influence over that which is beyond the pregnant woman's power. At a time when the nauseous and often salivating woman is so preoccupied with orality, food offers a means of modifying her symptoms. In addition, it is a way of making contact with the baby, or affecting its growth.

Cravings may have symbolic meanings, based on unconscious magical equations. Superstitious ideas abound, such as strong or savoury foods to fortify the baby, rich ones to ensure its wealth or cleverness, or milk to promote lactation, and so on.

Many folk beliefs reflect the idea that the food a woman eats will directly mark or affect the baby's growth or appearance. For instance, the Middle Eastern association of white foods with bone production or pale complexion; the European avoidance of strawberries for fear of birthmarks; the North African avoidance of mishapen root vegetables for fear of deformities. In Hong Kong, many Chinese women abstain from eating snake soup, which will produce a 'scaly'-skinned baby, or tea, which will produce a brown-skinned one. In many countries, rabbit meat is avoided because of associations with harelip. Some dietary restrictions are part of an elaborate belief system about health being dependent on balanced forces, such as hot and cold foods. Food taboo recommendations may be geared to the baby's development, or aim to increase the pregnant woman's health or ease her labour. For the pregnant woman, the main symbolic property of food is as a bridge between outer and inner worlds, between herself and the embryo. Food can represent a means of contact or influence. Cravings may be attributed to the pregnancy or seen as expressions of the baby, or as a complex means of identification with the fetus. A woman may use her cravings to gain extra cossetting or proof of love, as in the anecdotal stories about the husband's attempt to obtain out-of-season fruit. Sometimes the special 'treat' may be intended not for her, but for the baby.

Like cigarettes or alcohol or drugs, where readily available, food can be used by an expectant mother as a means to underline her bodily autonomy, despite the inmate's 'takeover bid'; or as a defence to fortify her against the 'invader'; or as a filler to close up an emotional gap within her. Women with eating disorders such as compulsive eating, bulimia or anorexic tendencies, are particularly vulnerable during pregnancy. Unhealthy intake and substance abuse may be used to control, test, or punish the baby, and a disturbed woman may relish her power to starve, harm, or inflict suffering on the fetus as a despised aspect of her baby self.

Primal Cavity

In many women, the emotional and physical upheaval of pregnancy reactivates childhood imagery about the interior of the body, such as the idea of a single internal space in which all the organs are interconnected, arousing a fantasy that the baby might be contaminated, or become entangled. A related fear is that when the 'plug' is removed in labour, the contents of the body will come gushing out; or as the cord is pulled after the birth, it will yank out everything else with it. This particular fear is heightened at times of precarious self-esteem and indefinite boundaries, or when the body interior is felt to be harbouring the true self, which is protected from the world: 'I'm terrified of blood tests. When they puncture my skin, I feel I might come pouring out. It's as if there's a vacuum inside and my inner self is liquid – as soft as the yolk of a soft-boiled egg which I've never, ever eaten', says Rachel early on in pregnancy.

Early bodily memories are revived with the physical treatment of her pregnant body. Fear of internal examinations may be related to inhibitions about genital exposure or terrors of being manhandled abusively:

> 'I can't bear the thought of internal examinations', says Polly, newly pregnant. 'Last time they were so painful, so rough, detached. I tried dissociating as if I wasn't there while lying there with my legs up in the air and that hostile intrusion by a rubberized hand – but it still affected my feelings in intercourse for months. I couldn't bear to be touched.'

When the body is conceptualized as a tube, orifices become interconnected. Grabbed by feelings of panic and choking, as her throat closed up, Rachel had the fantasy as she lay on the examination couch that the doctor's hand would reappear through her mouth.

Some women may employ defensive splitting to ensure internal 'partitions', with stocks and provisions kept in one compartment, separated from waste products. Others are concerned about the mixup of internal stuff – masticated food, urine, faeces, blood, sperm, amniotic fluid, milk, and flatus. To some, the body interior may seem a friendly and comfortable place; others imagine a dark, claustrophobic labyrinth cramping the pinioned fetus, or an empty void with a lonely fetus tethered to a placenta, spinning in empty space.

In an unhappy relationship the unborn child may have been mentally conceived to fulfil a role. He or she may be designated saviour, repairer, new start, proof of love, scapegoat, pawn, pleasurer. The list is endless – the disappointment inevitable. Sometimes, to differentiate the imaginary baby from the real one to come, the bump is given a nominal tag such as Popeye or Geronimo – a name that will not be used after the birth. Naming the fetus gives licence to engage in fanciful narratives while, paradoxically, locating the unseen fetus in the world of real social exchanges: 'Let's take a banana when we go to the theatre. You know how Matilda loves them.'

Technological innovations have disturbed the mysteriousness of the primordial process of unleashed fantasy. Prenatal knowledge of the baby's features and its sex, through sonography or amniocentesis, may puncture the bubble of imagining, as parents begin relating to a sexed individual. Fibre-optic photography enables us to see the baby in action in the womb environment, and how she or he responds to different stimuli. Furthermore, what has now been demonstrated beyond doubt is that the fetus is aware of subtle changes in both the internal and external environment, discriminating in response to physical experiences (dark-light, movements, sounds, tastes, touch); social stimulation (conversation, singing, dancing, music, stroking); and emotional changes (in maternal hormones, metabolism, heart rate, moods). Even in the womb, the human baby is being influenced by the specific culture of his mother's environment. He or she is a complex and competent being, who seeks meaning and responds in a way which makes sense. Pregnancy is a time of conduction: like impulses from nerve endings sparking across neurones in electrical discharge, transmissions occur across uterine boundaries. The baby is growing to know a world beyond the womb through the impact of maternal biorhythms, hormonal influences, and her patterns of movement, sleep, and intake, and, indirectly, through her activities. As mothers have suspected throughout time, in ways mild and intense, properties of each pregnant woman's emotional and material world infiltrate the womb.

Three in the Bed

With confirmation of pregnancy, sex – no longer simply play-time nor a purposeful propagatory act between two partners — hooks into another sphere where three interact. To some women, the baby, conceived by making love, is in itself the essence of love, or verification of it. To others, conception signifies possession of a working sexual body, or evidence of femininity, virility, or potency, and pregnancy may arouse resentment or envy in the man, or discontentment in the woman, seeming not a blissful prerogative but an exhausting process from which males are unfairly spared.

Intercourse may subtly change from a recreative or procreative activity to one of celebration of mutual creation or expression of separate bodily experiences. Conception of a wanted baby often heightens tenderness in intercourse, bringing the couple closer together as they enter their new state as expectant parents, freed from the shadows of disapproval and doubt. They may experience a rejuvenation of sexual desire now that a planned pregnancy is finally achieved – or, ironically in the case of an unexpected one, when fate has decreed they no longer need to be anxious about pregnancy occurring.

Sexuality itself is replete with mysteries of the primal scene – the original parents' secret activities. When conception signifies entry into a forbidden zone, lovemaking may be enhanced or inhibited according to the emotional charge of the underlying unconscious fantasy. The intimate physical connection between lovers draws its electric power from the intermingling of childhood desires and mature concerns. A playground for suspension of limitations and dividedness, it also underscores male and female differences – especially during pregnancy.

Submission to orgasmic fusion and oblivion is often associated with the idea of re-entering the womb. During pregnancy – when someone actually *does* reside in the womb – this fantasy is complicated by the mixture of inhibiting awareness of an intruder, and/or identification with the fetus *in utero*. The privacy of a twosome is intercepted by the presence of a third. A pregnant dyad may oscillate between feeling that the pregnancy enriches their intimate relationship and experiencing a sense of invasion, imagining the fetus occupying the place of the penis, or spying on their copulation from within. In exhibitionistic sexual fantasies, the audience component often becomes invested in the fetus; or the baby may symbolize the rival, the baby-self, the split-off villain, the voyeuristic child, the incestuous progeny. Or the pregnant woman, now mother-to-be, may acquire an aura of the forbidden maternal object. Complex issues of possessiveness feature in their relationship, as pregnancy raises the question of who her inner body belongs to: herself, her baby, or her man.

Pregnancy alters a woman's internal experience of her sexuality, as her spontaneous responses are shaped by unfamiliar bodily sensations and hormonal experiences, as well as by her psychic experience of the pregnancy. Her body is no longer her own. She is more than the sum of herself, no longer a single, unitary being: she contains a growing part of her mate, while he remains as physically indivisible and separate as he has been since birth. Physiologically and psychologically, he is unchanged while pregnancy influences every sphere of her bodily and psychic experience, including sex: 'I'm not sure sex would establish "us" again in renewed closeness. We're very different now because I'm wrapped up in what's going on inside me and feel so bloody awful; I've retreated inwards, while he's still on the surface.'

Changes in a woman's circulatory system during pregnancy include increased vascularity in the entire pelvic area, changing her capacity for sexual tension by enhancing the frequency and intensity of orgasm. Increased hormonal production influences the elasticity and relaxation of smooth muscles, ligaments, and soft-connective tissue. Profuse vaginal secretions alternate with unusual dryness, affecting her receptivity to erotic stimulation. All of these, plus the natural endorphin-induced sense of wellbeing and intensified nipple and clitoral sensitivity, may contribute to heightened experience of sexuality. Some pregnant women find this frightening, feeling anxious about unleashing a hitherto restrained passionate aspect of themselves.

During the first trimester a woman is aware not only of the physical changes but also of the new and strange sense of her body as a vessel, containing prime matter. Both she and her partner may feel concerned about the effect of intercourse on the tender embryo, fearing it may cause a miscarriage or harm the baby in some way. The fetus is in fact well protected from damage or infection, and sex cannot dislodge it. Nevertheless, anxieties may persist well into pregnancy:

'I'm completely disinterested in sex. I just don't want anything. I feel physically content, as if the baby must have plugged a deep physical need. I feel cut off, and don't want anything from outside. I suppose I feel penetration might not be pleasant for a child – all that battering – and I hold back from orgasm because I'm afraid of uterine contractions. But most of all I'm perturbed because I have no desire. I don't want us distanced. Pregnancy has brought us closer together, yet it has also greatly increased our separateness – I'm the one who is growing the baby and he has done his bit . . .'

Shared Differences

The partners have become intensely different. Even at rest she is an active generator; even alone she is no longer on her own. The male partner may feel excluded; the female invaded or exploited. She has morning sickness and a thickening waist, he remains unchanged. She has direct contact with the baby, he feels left out. Deep resentments, which often remain unconscious, may surface during lovemaking, creating physical tension and unspoken conflicts between the partners. The male may feel rejected: 'Now she's pregnant, she's discarded me sexually. Sometimes I feel like a spider's mate that is consumed after fertilization.'

No Man's Land

In his wish to contribute to the baby's development, an expectant father may unconsciously equate ejaculation with feeding, imagining he is watering the fetus to encourage growth, or nourishing it with milky sperm. He may also feel newly aroused: his mate's burgeoning fertility seems exciting and magnificently attractive. Other men find their partner's pregnant body strangely undesirable, and feel defensively remote or disturbed by the sense of her becoming a mother, and hence, Oedipally forbidden. On a more primitive level, she has become the source, the secret mysterious place from whence he himself originated – the whole from which he was split off and divided.

For the man, the body he now makes love to is no longer the prepregnancy one which conceived his child: 'I married a sports car, but overnight she's turned into a bus.' Her smell, the feel of her skin, the texture of her hair are all subtly altered. Her shape changes before his very eyes, as breasts expand, veins protrude, waist is lost, and belly swells. A man may feel very tender towards this woman who is carrying his child, increasing sexual contact as a means of expressing his love for her.

In this transitional state, unconscious fantasies flourish. Awestruck by her creative powers, or feeling redundant now that conception has occurred, or identifying with his impregnating sperm, a partner may be fearful of being sucked back into the closed womb. A common fantasy is that the baby may grab hold of his penis during intercourse. Deeply disturbing fantasies, and envy of the female internal treasure and/or fear of the retaliating Oedipal father are often presented in dreams.

In later pregnancy, although the male partner may feel more relaxed because the baby's robustness seems assured, its increased liveliness can be sexually inhibiting. The sense of a fetus always watching can lead to loss of erection in a man who feels persecuted externally, or by his own internal demanding baby. Unconscious phallic sadism may incapacitate the man with fears of hurting the fetus or the pregnant woman with his swordlike penis, resulting in temporary impotence. In cases of unresolved envy of the female partner's creativity, partners flare up with gastric or genital symptoms which prevent intercourse, or graphically express contamination fears or anxieties about the untouchable woman. In other cases, shaky masculine identification may manifest in envy and appropriation of antenatal care and birth plans, or macho dominance-displays of verbal and/or physical violence, sexual coercion, and even rape.

A woman may feel passionately sexual during this phase of her pregnancy, while her partner is inhibited by his unconscious anxieties. Alienation may grow if they differ in the intensity of their sexual desires and are unable to voice their feelings to each other. Either may feel rejected or unvalued by the other. Sensitivity about her changed appearance may contribute to a woman's sense of unattractiveness, which she feels is confirmed by her partner's sexual disinterest. He may cautiously be awaiting signs of encouragement from her, afraid of inflicting himself upon her, as if they were the pre-pregnant lovers of old.

In the second trimester, uterine contractions during orgasm increase, and the post-orgasmic phase of uterine relaxation is slower. Some women feel released from sexual inhibitions, relishing newfound sensuality, and ironically, freedom from previous concern about conception. Some women experience greater sexual excitement, and the amplification of orgasm may cause somatic-alarm and/or fears of triggering miscarriage. (Reviewing recent research, obstetrician Wendy Savage has concluded that no harm can come to the baby from sexual intercourse.)

Mid-pregnancy is the period when the majority of women feel physically most comfortable. Towards the end of pregnancy, when her body feels cumbersome and weighed down, a woman may be less inclined to have sex, although some continue feeling inordinately aroused throughout the latter part of pregnancy as well.

Warmth can find many forms of expression. Sexual activity is by no means the sole indicator of emotional closeness, and erotic pleasure need not involve penetration. As the 'bump' grows larger, and the reclining woman feels like a beached whale, motivation to find new ways of expressing their affection may serendipitously invigorate an expectant couple's lovemaking.

Accessing Feminine Mysteries

Now that the interior of her body has become galvanized into operation, it gathers mysteriousness rather than dispelling the enigma: 'This ripple takes over your body as you're standing by the sink washing up. Not an interference, but a communion, a miracle; a miracle, awesome beyond understanding. If I stop to think about it, it scrambles my mind.'

To the woman on the cold end of the probing speculum, internal examinations by the doctor, however unpleasant, signify an awaited message from the interior. She wants to know whether her womb is a creative, life-giving place. Blood pressure, scans, and urine tests are treated by the pregnant woman as part ritual, part revelation. Her antenatal visits are rites of passage, an affirmation of the quality of her inner manufacturing activity.

Technology provides a magical entrée to a hidden world, offering the intensely arousing experience of actually seeing her baby through ultrasound, observing him or her moving about, possibly even being given a video of the scan. Seeing the baby's activities, or even the features on the little face, and imagining the interior of her womb as the baby's home may assist prenatal bonding. In some instances, however, the number of professionals involved, their intrusiveness, and insensitivity to her emotional experience and the stress involved can actually increase rather than reduce anxiety.

Some parents feel disturbed by the Pandora's box of prenatal screening, arousing their anger at impossible choices, and introducing new worries about the effects of the tests. Along with increased familiarity of the real baby, there may be a sense of being cheated out of a period of free-floating fantasy. As ultrasound and amniocentesis provide information about the baby's sex, expectant parents may feel resentment at having to make choices; feeling compelled to know the baby's sex if the doctors do, they may feel deprived of surprise on the day of the birth.

Other expectant parents are anxious and in need of reassurance. Sometimes the simple experience of listening to the metronomic vigour of the baby's heartbeat can reinforce their optimism. Similarly, rather than treating her as an inert container, a professional's respect for a mother-to-be's awareness of her baby, or a warm confirmation that the baby is lucky to have her for a mother, often do more to allay anxieties and self-doubts than any tests.

Not all technological innovations are helpful or innocuous. We are now aware of the dangers of X-rays, and of various drugs such as Thalidomide, thought at the time to be beneficial to pregnant women. Not all antenatal screening procedures are informative, and some, like glucose tolerance tests, are deemed of unproven value, and likely to introduce unnecessary anxiety and unwarranted interventions. Given the drawbacks, we may ask why some women not only comply with routine screening, but often seek out further examinations.

On an unconscious level, the questions which preoccupy a pregnant woman in her search for information are the primordial feminine mysteries of containment, formation, preservation, and transformation. Psychologically, containment of her fears and emotional upheaval echo the containment of another inside her body. Faced with the enormity of her creative responsibility, doubts arise about her capacity to form a viable, healthy baby. Wondering how her body will know what to do, she worries whether she can rely on it to accomplish the magical process of gestation – to transform the invisible fertilized egg into an embryo, which could grow into a real, viable baby. And even if it does, will she be allowed to keep the child?

She is concerned with the issue of preservation: keeping her baby secure within her, protected from external and internal dangers. Preoccupation with such age-old mysteries is personal and practical. On a mundane level, she wonders how to continue her active life yet sustain the baby's growth, nourishing it and guarding it from hazards during gestation and unseen forces during the labour. Can she ensure her own wellbeing while maintaining a balanced ambiance inside her? Can she prevent it from falling out, or dissolving into nothing? Will she keep the baby happy, willing to stay inside until term? Pre-term births are often interpreted by the mother as a rejection, or a judgement by the baby on inhospitable conditions within.

She is concerned about the baby's normality, but also what the baby will think of hers. This baby, emerging from within, knows everything buried inside her, and could reveal its secrets to those around her. Can the baby withstand her internal badness? Can he or she benefit from her goodness? As for that extraordinary mystery of transformation, can she achieve the multiple miracle of turning a tiny seed into a fetus, a pregnancy into a baby, bodily fluids into milk, and herself into a mother? These are a few of the enigmas on which women around the world seek guidance – employing any magical, traditional or scientific means at their disposal.

3
The Placental Paradigm

'The cords of all link back, strandentwining cable of all flesh
. . . Spouse and helpmate of Adam Kadmon: Heva, Eve. She
has no navel. Gaze. Belly without blemish, bulging big, a
buckler of taut vellum, no, whiteheaped corn, orient and im-
mortal, standing from everlasting to everlasting. Womb of sin.

Wombed in sin darkness I was too, made not begotten. By
them, the man with my voice and my eyes and a ghostwoman
with ashes on her breath. They clasped and sundered, did the
coupler's will. From before the ages He willed me and now
may not will me away or ever. . . .'

James Joyce, *Ulysses*

Throughout the generations, each of us – male and female – has
begun life inside a maternal body. Our first impressions were the
walls of the womb, the taste of amniotic fluid, and the muffled
sound of a female voice. For most of us, a woman wielded power
over our infantile helplessness, the source of joy and anguish.
Pregnancy is our sensual bedrock, and this state revitalizes primitive experiences in the woman, herself turned container.
Shadows from the past permeate her present, and as her body
recaptures the maternal stance, her inner world is galvanized into
emotional upheaval.

In her interchanging identification with the woman who bore
her, and herself as bearer of her baby, a pregnant woman may
conceptualize a daisy-chain of cords linking her back, navel to
navel, through the maternal line to the woman with no navel.
Most expectant mothers know that the cord connecting them has
a double function: it conveys nutrients to the baby, while removing fetal waste products to be cleared through her own systems.
For better or for worse, for the duration of the pregnancy they
are a yoked dyad. According to her mood, the mother may focus
on the positive or negative aspects of this two-way, give-and-
take process, seeing herself as a passive container, a bountiful
provider, a stingy hoarder, a damaging poisoner, or an exploited

hostess. By the same token, she may at times imagine her baby as an innocent guest, a depleting parasite, sapping her energies; an intrusive alien, contaminating her insides; an internal saboteur, who may attack and damage her; a confined prisoner, a vulnerable being, or a friendly inmate. The cord that links them may thus be imagnied as a two-way conduit, envisioned by some as a source of special joy: 'This is the closest we'll ever be – exchanging our very life-blood'; and to others threatening retaliatory persecution: 'When I think of the umbilical cord,' says another pregnant woman afraid to feel angry 'it's as if what goes out of me will come shooting back.'

Although books on pregnancy pay little attention to the placenta, to the pregnant woman it often has great emotional significance. It may be imagined as an organ she has grown especially for the baby, or one that the prudent fetus has brought along to feed itself. Depending on her perspective, the placenta may symbolize her bountifulness or insufficiency; fetal greed or their symbiotic dependence.

In the absence of knowledge about her baby, the womb becomes a receptacle for the woman's fantasies, wishes, fears, and hopes. Her fantasy baby is woven out of the stuff of her dreams and her internal view of herself. Like an imaginary friend, it is a mirage acquiring shape and solidity from borrowed narratives and emotional residues of her inner story. Throughout pregnancy, fluctuations occur in the expectant mother's attachment to her fetus. These may be determined by her health, the emotional support she receives, demands by other dependents, and, above all, the internal resources on which she draws. Nevertheless, from studying pregnant women daily over the course of a pregnancy, or in some cases several gestations, I have found that despite day-by-day variations, most women evolve an attitude of mind towards the fetus and themselves, ascribing positive and negative attributes and value judgments to each.

The placental paradigm is a model I have elaborated to schematize these emotional permutations. It focuses on the mother's imagined interchange between herself and her inmate, the two-way process she envisages, conveying substances as well as receiving and filtering them.

Depending on whether the mother deems the exchange between herself and her fetus benign or harmful, she will erect or dismantle imaginary barriers between them. How she views their interaction stems from unconscious concepts of the fetus and her self-image as good or dangerous. Most pregnant women's fantasies fluctuate throughout the pregnancy between these various positions according to their moods and symptoms. In general, however, each woman tends to gravitate towards one or other stance in accordance with her emotional orientation to this particular pregnancy and habitual modes of defence.

The placental paradigm shows how the quality of a pregnant woman's self-image and feelings about her unborn baby can influence her emotional experience of the gestation, the postnatal encounter and her behaviour as a mother. In her mind, co-existence is possible if the expectant mother is able to tolerate her ambivalence towards the pregnancy. She then can allow herself to think of the baby, too, as a mixture: sometimes innocently growing inside her, unaware of her existence; at other times, wilfully nudging her or ruthlessly tiring her out. It is likely that such a woman will be able to continue after the birth to see herself as a good-enough mother to a good-enough baby.

Conversely, the woman who idealizes the pregnant exchange, regarding both herself and her baby as only positive, will blossom by denying any negative aspects, indulging in fantasies of mutually enriching, pooled resources. This expectant mother not only sees herself as bountiful provider, but luxuriates by proxy in the paradisal state of her imagined fetus. Unless she mourns the passing of their exclusive intimacy, she may try to re-establish it postnatally, with herself as all-embracing emotional container in a symbiotic merger that, once again, denies any imperfections.

The pregnant woman who feels internally persecuted by her fetus – prey to a dangerous being greedily feeding off her resources, or polluting her with its waste products – will feel compelled to establish a mental barrier that enables her to protect some good things inside herself from exploitation. This may take the form of emotional detachment, doing her own thing and refusing to allow her thoughts to be taken over by the fetus. Or she may eat for two in order to counter the anxiety of being internally devoured or sucked dry by the fetus; or drink lots to flush out the baby's waste products. She may attribute symptoms such as flatulence, heartburn, or constipation to the baby's malign influence or to her defences against it: 'I feel as though my whole body is in rebellion against this hijacking.'

Conversely, when a pregnant woman feels it is she who is a bad influence on her vulnerable, good baby, she may constantly resort to superstitious behaviour to avoid seepage of her bad emotions or habits: 'Without a drink I keep crashing up against the fascist in me', says a desperate alcoholic who has referred herself for therapy. 'But with it I endanger the baby, so I have to spend all day trying to think positive thoughts to compensate for reaching for the bottle.' Once born, the baby who has been inside her and knows her badness from within may be at times experienced as tolerant or resilient, but at other times accusatory or damning. She may alternate between acceptance and guilt:

> 'My little boy is so skinny and still doesn't sleep well', says the mother of a three-year-old. 'I'm convinced it's because I smoked when pregnant with him. He's very tough, but it haunts me, this feeling that something is wrong and I caused it.'

The pregnant woman who is chronically insecure about her own value may seek constant reassurance not only that she does have some good resources, but of the baby's capacity to withstand her badness. As one such pregnant woman says:

> 'Sometimes when I panic, I feel blown to pieces as if my whole body will fall apart and nothing can keep me together. I'm afraid the baby could be blown out or poisoned. It's so cold and bad inside me – I know, I've lived like this for years. I've soothed myself with food and dope, keeping my craziness to myself. But this baby, it's right in there in the middle of it all – it can't get away . . .'

If both she and the baby are conceptualized as dangerous to each other – a fantasy exacerbated by Rhesus incompatibility – the woman may resolve her dilemma by attempting to erect an impermeable barrier between them, refusing to be involved with the pregnancy at all. Another may become anorexic, refusing to feed the baby, and in her mind punishing her own mother who deprived her. Or, resolving that each will go their own way, she may step up her activities to prove their mutual independence. Similarly, the expectant woman may refuse to make any concessions to her pregnancy, or continue to smoke, drink, or take drugs – not as a test of the baby's tolerance, as in the above cases, but to demonstrate her resentment at its interference in her life: 'I'm not impressed with all this pampering business. Pregnancy's normal so you just get on with normal life.' Postnatally, unless the mother has had therapeutic support or gets a baby who has unusual capacities to override her indifference, guilty overcompensation or rancour, supplementary care giving is essential.

The Mother as Container

There is a psychoanalytic idea of a mother as a 'container'. Wilfred Bion proposed that, ideally, mothers, who are the recipients of their baby's anxieties 'contain' these until the infant has established a notion of his or her own inner space in which to keep them. A 'good' mother will hold the baby's unthinkable thoughts, mentally digest them through her 'maternal reverie', and then convey the mitigated emotions so they can be safely taken back by the infant. I am suggesting that a paradigm for this mothering process exists long before the baby is born. The pregnant mother is already serving as a container for her baby, and through the give and take of the placental process, is both nourishing and metabolizing his or her waste products in her own body. The degree to which she feels threatened by the baby's 'poisons' or her own destructive forces, reduces her enjoyment of their placental linkage during pregnancy and receptivity to an emotional dialogue postnatally.

Much of the expectant mother's unconscious configurations are coloured by her own emotional framework and the place of the child in her psychic reality. Identifying with both mother and baby, some women idealize the mother/baby fusion, defending against ambivalence by investing the baby with endearing aspects of their own imagined baby-selves, and/or glorifying the fetus and the fantasy of a symbiotic merger with a generous, benevolent mother. Others imbue the baby with the unruly aspects of themselves that they feel they have outgrown, or with the repudiated facets of their own internal worlds – which may include repressed incestuous wishes, or experiences of abuse.

The more tolerant a woman is of her own mixed feelings, and those of her own mother, and the more accepting she is of the babyish and childlike aspects of herself, the greater the likelihood of her owning these, rather than splitting them off and projecting them into the baby with whom she unconsciously identifies. She will then not have to go to great lengths to defend against the threats she feels lurking within herself or attributes to the baby. This in turn enhances her capacity to be in touch with what she is experiencing emotionally, rather than having to maintain elaborate mechanisms of defence, such as altruism, idealization, disavowal, or detachment, in order to protect herself from awareness of the dialectic of love and hate, child and adult, sophisticated and primitive processes, which exist in us all.

Placental Paradigm

Mother	Baby	Psychic Interchange
±	±	ambivalent coexistence
+	+	idealized exchange
+	−	mother's barrier against 'parasitic' baby
−	+	mother feels dangerous to vulnerable baby
+/−	0	bipolar conflict: good/bad splitting; baby=non-entity

As a metaphor this paradigm has proved more apt than I thought when first proposing it in 1989. In recent months, evolutionary biologists have established that, since only half the baby's genes come from the mother, the genetic interests of fetus and pregnant woman are not always identical and at times, an internal tug-of-war rages over resources, altering the mother's biochemistry to accommodate the needs of her inmate. Since a woman's view of herself and unconscious configurations of her baby come to influence postnatal interaction, pregnant women who feel troubled by their inability to engage with the idea of having a baby or feel persecuted by it, may seek psychotherapeutic help to foster a resolution of internal conflicts before the two-way interactive process begins at birth.

4
The Place of Paternity

Caesarean over, as the doctor takes the baby back to cut the cord, the father peeps over the screen. Alphonse, his pet fetus, has been swapped for a girl! The child he is handed isn't the one he's held in mind and played imaginary games with all these months. This little scrap, her eyes screwed tight against the bright lights, is female like her mother. His son, his male stake in the future, his claim to connectedness has evaporated with the appearance of a penis-less newborn.

As a major operation begins to dock the wrapped baby on to the nipple, the new father stands by, throat congested with unshed tears of joy, impotence, frustration, and relief, feeling like an intruder in the female scene. All he wants to do is to unwrap the baby and stick it under his shirt, skin to skin, and laze about crooning and babbling to smooth her way into the noisy harsh ward. But he is overlooked in the nurses' efforts, and anyway, he's afraid she'll think he smells wrong . . .

Faced with the female prerogatives of pregnancy and birth, the male partner finds himself, as did his father, struggling to establish his own contribution. Even at rest, his partner's pregnant body sustains the baby growing within her, while he has to work to maintain contact, and to find his place within the productive sphere. After the birth, too, the father's link remains an act of faith, based on trust and social acceptance.

Throughout time, in most societies women have been primarily defined by their procreative and maternal roles, while men have had to construct masculine identities in counter-identification to female mothering. With technological advances in genetic fingerprinting, which can determine the identity of the biological father, womb surrogacy, and gamete donation not only of sperm but of ovum – or its *in vitro* fertilization outside the body – some of the asymmetry between mother and father has been reduced. With increasing acceptance of single parenting and cohabitation of unmarried couples, the practice of paternal acknowledgement of offspring by the man bequeathing his surname is no longer sufficient for paternity. Fathers are having to engage in parental activities to earn the paternal position previously nominally granted to them. Fathering, like mothering, is fast becoming a continuous verb. Conversely, men seem to be beginning to be more possessive of their paternal rights, and even sperm donors have been known to demand access to the fathered child.

Unlike his pregnant partner who carries a visible bulge, the expectant father may feel, and indeed often is, left out and overlooked by friends and health care professionals. Escaping the physical discomforts of pregnancy and birth, he forgoes the pleasure of experiencing internal life, and may feel jealous of the intimacy his partner shares with their baby. (Interestingly, expectant parents of twins may both feel excluded from the intimacy which the babies enjoy with each other in the womb.) Tactile contact is made through his partner's skin, and as he tries to fondle the little body, or feels the impact of its movements, he perhaps cannot help but wonder what it must feel like to be experiencing them from within.

Envy by the man of the woman's capacity to grow their baby is not uncommon. Freud's descriptions of 'Little Hans' and the 'Wolf Man' refer to the boy's early desire to have a baby in identification with his mother as well as a wish to be born of the father, to be sexually satisfied by him, and to present him with a child. This culminates in a fantasy of getting inside the mother's womb in order to replace her in intercourse with father. During his partner's pregnancy, disturbing infantile fantasies and deep-seated envy of her capacities and of the baby inside her, may re-emerge in the male.

Couvade

Couvade is a cultural ritual facilitating the father's acknowledgement of paternity, portraying in symbolic form his commitment to the baby. In some societies couvade is intended to protect the woman or her unborn baby from demons or evil spirits by diverting their attention to the father. Some early psychoanalysts and anthropologists recognized the father's unconscious hostility towards his partner and/or baby underlying formalized couvade rituals. Yet in addition to providing an emotional outlet for the man's mixed feelings, on an intrapsychic level couvade also is a form of unconscious identification with both woman and fetus, enabling the man to deflect his rivalry and ambivalence through creativity, and to gain sympathy by arousing public attention.

In industrialized societies, in the absence of formal rituals, symptom formation may replace couvade, offering the expectant father a means of repudiating his hostility while bearing punishment for it. Psychosomatic illnesses may also express his envy of the woman and early fantasies about his own capacity to bear babies. Symptoms provide a means of gaining paternal recognition and care by professionals and others, as well as escape from responsibilities, and respite for contemplation possibly involving time off work.

Research suggests that as many as half the population of expectant fathers develop some symptoms relating to pregnancy during the course of gestation. Various studies have confirmed a preponderance of hypochondriacal obsessions among expectant fathers, which may be a means of unconsciously transferring the focus of attention to their own bodies.

Some psychosomatic symptoms such as morning sickness and weight gain in fathers-to-be directly mimic pregnancy or center on discomfort or pain in sympathy with those the female will have to bear. Others are precipitated by pregnancy but are more diffuse, such as palpitations, acute anxiety, and so on. A more sublimated expression of envy may manifest in the partners, as in over-solicitous involvement in and control of the intake and bodily functions of the pregnant woman and her birth preparation, or establishment of a creative project simulating gestation or competing with pregnancy, possibly even timed to coincide with the birth. In cases where the man is anxious about early fatherhood, his 'project' may be geared to absenting him from the birth, or the first threatening postnatal days or weeks.

Taken to extremes – as opposed to occasional sympathetic reactions – psychosomatic symptoms indicate that bypassing thought and feeling, the body is being used regressively to manifest old conflicts. Seeking treatment by male medical authority figures may express submission, a compromise of identification and/or competitiveness with the maternal love object, rather than risking masculine rivalry with a fearsome Oedipal father.

In addition to symptoms simulating childbearing, some seem to relate to unconscious identification with the fetus:

'I dreamed I was sitting on the sofa bed and my mother hardly said a word to me. I felt impotently furious. She took up all the room . . . she's always taken me for granted and ignored me, leaving me just enough to keep alive. I've only been given the bare necessities for survival, never enough to go and come and be in the world.' Reported an expectant father after an asthma attack.

The Father's Father

The experience of awaiting a first baby activates intense emotions, as a man begins to move into the place of the father, displacing his own father into the grandparents' generation. About to become a parent, awaiting a child triggers a man's re-evaluation of the past as child to his own parents. Tender memories of being carried in his father's arms or triumphantly perched on his shoulders may jostle with images of his father's face distorted with brutal rage. A bittersweet mixture of swirling emotions converge in recalled and unconscious experiences of father-son separations and reunions, cold indifference, or a yearning for warmth.

Painful reverberations of being his Oedipal mother's son rather than lover may also re-emerge. Phallic pride in his capacity to procreate mingle with old feelings of intense rivalry relating to his father's exclusive privilege to make love and babies. How this basic conflict has been resolved will determine the man's attitude towards this pregnancy:

- Whether helped by a loving father (see Layland) the boy was able to identify with him, yet relinquish his impossible desires.
- Whether he circumvented the issue by remaining identified with his birth-giving mother (thus denying the limitations of his own gender) or by desiring not mother, but father.
- Whether he failed to enter into the arena at all, living out a fantasy life with his mother deprived of the challenge of a father's emotional or physical presence.

Revision of the past during pregnancy can in some men bring about about a reappraisal of internal relationships, resulting in resynthesis into the sense of self. In most men the process of transition to fatherhood takes place in dreams, day reveries, and conscious memories. It is often played out in reality with his father, or with other important male figures and mentors.

Some expectant fathers are able to grasp the significance of these experiences and work through the feelings associated with them; others deflect them from consciousness, relying on action rather than thought. If mature affirmation is achieved, and paternal attributes are recognized as well as faults, the man will find himself, like each male generation before him, in ascendance as his father's powers decline.

The Expectant Father

The majority of studies have focused on women during pregnancy. It is only in recent years that expectant fathers have become the focus in their own right.

An Israeli study by Gerzi and Berman compared fifty-one expectant fathers with fifty-one married men without children. The former rated significantly higher on overall anxiety and tension, and in projective tests indicated stronger Oedipal preoccupations and dependency needs, sibling rivalry, and equation of the expected baby with an envied younger sibling. Clinical interviews with some of the expectant fathers revealed ambivalence, guilt, infantile fantasies, feminine identifications, castration fears, and considerable defence mechanisms.

Another recent focus has been on the developmental shifts which occur in the resynthesized sense of self of expectant fathers. Various studies by American psychoanalysts (such as Cath, Gurwitt, Ross, and Herzog) have found that awareness of their life-creating forces encourages men towards reconciliation with their own fathers. Men who fail to sort out their relationships with their fathers during pregnancy become progressively less able to find an internal male mentor to protect them from feminine identification. In some men residual 'father hunger', due to physical or emotional absence while the boy was growing up, leads to mid-pregnancy pursuit of males and maleness through bisexual adventures or extramarital affairs. Similarly, a recent study at the Institute of Psychiatry in London has confirmed the father's relationship with his own father as being the single most significant factor in postnatal male mental illness (see Lovestone and Kumar).

In my clinical experience, pregnancy can jolt stymied internal relationships out of their stable compromise positions, resulting either in protective rigidification, or easing up of defences. For some expectant fathers, public proof of virility affects lifelong habits in relation to father figures – freeing blocked creativity that has been held back in deference to authority, or ending patterns of cocky rebelliousness as a man becomes better able to tolerate uncertainty and ambivalence.

In either case, an awareness of how far he and his partner have come coupled with how far they have yet to go may turn the pregnancy into a journey of self-discovery accompanied by solid confidence and flourishing initiative. Others, unable to achieve a fruitful reconciliation with an internal, forbidding father image, may begin to manifest psychosomatic symptoms or sexual, social, or work difficulties as unresolved Oedipal conflicts are revived.

If the pregnancy is unconsciously experienced as a transgression, old, irrational fears of primitive retribution – castration, or being sucked back into the womb – may result in panic states, or a variety of activities to relieve or avoid anxiety. Thus, an expectant father might counteract fears of impotence and passivity with promiscuity, or reckless activity such as dangerous driving or madcap adventures. He may avoid intercourse with his burgeoning wife by seeking a lover on the grounds of concern for her health, or have recurrent infections which prevents their intimacy. Authoritative internal father figures may be appeased by reverting to an unchallenging little-boy-like attitude towards his boss and elders, or passive surrender, inviting homosexual encounters with older men. Alternatively, in a desperate attempt to prove his threatened masculinity, he may become belligerent and challenging towards representatives of paternal authority, or over-possessive of his partner.

A recurrent theme in fathers-to-be is that of helpless resentment at having so little influence over such a momentous process. Sometimes a division of labour emerges during pregnancy: she gets on with forming the baby, while he does the 'mental' work – worrying for both – thereby relieving her of the necessity to be anxious. It may reflect his realistic concern, or neurotic preoccupation about the baby's growth. In some couples, the man's excessive worry may be the flip-side of her denial of concern – particularly if she eats erratically, smokes, drinks, or behaves in a way he feels endangers his baby's wellbeing.

'I've become like my mother, pervading the house with reverberations of doom and disaster because Elaine's so damn blasé about this pregnancy. She's got high blood pressure but never rests and keeps on eating salt, and won't for a minute consider it's any of my business what she's doing to our baby', says a man in therapy.

The expectant father's focus on her 'abusive' activities and generalized sense of foreboding may reflect his identification with the helplessness of the fetal recipient, as well as the powerlessness of his bystander status. Even in the absence of cause for concern, some fathers-to-be may become preoccupied with their partner's intake as one means of gaining control over the process of gestation. Others engage in obsessional rituals or superstitious behaviour in a vain attempt to exert magical power over the outcomes, since nothing they do seems to have an effect.

In extreme cases, unable to tolerate his secondary status, a man may resort to violence as a means of mitigating his anxiety and sense of being undermined. At this time when he feels his male authority is being eroded, or even usurped by her internal possession of a baby or imagined penis, verbal or physical abuse is intended to keep the woman in check, and remind her of who is boss. If she seems to have it all, and he is unable to sublimate his envy of her fullness and lifegiving capacity, an envious man may use destructive force to assert his own masculine power.

Already during pregnancy male partners in emotionally dependent relationships feel threatened by the baby's hold on the woman. Violence is an extreme bid to claim back the attention he feels has been stolen from him, which she now lavishes on the baby – as his mother's attention might have been focused on rival siblings. The target is not only the treacherous woman, but may be directed at her belly and the fetus.

Although these situations are often tolerated by couples as understandable, it is now well documented that violence in pregnancy can lead not only to miscarriages, prematurity, and low-birth-weight complications, but fetal abuse is a recognized antecedent to neonaticide or child abuse, while domestic violence is known to persist and escalate postnatally.

Paternal Contributions

Unlike traditional societies, which clearly define the tasks of an expectant father and the activities he must perform, Western society leaves the man to his own resources. A profusion of choices exist, ranging from full-scale participation in the pregnancy, birth, and baby care, to renunciation and avoidance of any feminine identification. Some fathers relegate the entire responsibility of the baby to the woman; others supplement the initial genetic contribution with emotional involvement throughout the pregnancy. Depending on his psychic reality and confidence in the process of growth, a man may utilize feminine identification with his early mother – not in competition with the woman, but to express nurturant, empathic aspects of his personality.

When a pregnant woman for unconscious reasons doubts her creative capacities, her partner's emotional envelopment may fill a maternal gap in her internal world. Conversely, his skepticism and internal conflicts can exacerbate her own, at times driving her to act out or disperse her anxiety through psychosomatic or addictive patterns. Her negative feelings about the fetus can be mitigated if he acknowledges his share in making the baby, or become exaggerated by his disavowal.

Labour

A fairly recent phenomenon is the pressure on fathers to participate in birth education classes, and to attend the labour and birth. To their surprise, many men find this to be a gruelling but exhilarating experience (see Greenberg), and look back with great pleasure: 'It was a profound once-in-a-lifetime moment when my son popped out – and I was there to see it!'

Presence at the birth may also play a part in priming protective emotional responses. Rosenblatts's studies on rats have illustrated that males who would normally eat the pups, not only do not do so if exposed to them soon after the birth, but actually develop maternalistic behaviour.

Birth highlights the bedrock difference between the sexes as no other situation can; it is a confrontation with the basic facts of life some men find intolerable. Fear of feeling like a spare part in a female world, of guilt at having put her through this painful experience while unable to share in it in any direct way may colour labour with a sense of personal shame or disturbing helplessness. When a couple can share their concern with each other, and discuss their respective wishes, even if these differ, they may arrive at an agreement that enables them both to protect their own emotional interests:

'I admit I felt somewhat churlish about refusing to accompany her during her ordeal, and selfish too, worrying about the effect it might have on me. So I was very relieved when she admitted it was better if I didn't come because she was afraid she'd be worrying about the effect on her of my being there.'

When a man decides to decline, his own desire to guard himself should be respected, although it is preferable to make an informed decision, as with hindsight some men regret not having been present at the birth of their child, and others who thought it might be alarming have not found it so.

Male anxieties tend to revolve around impotence in the face of her pain and being frightened and sickened by the intense emotional demands and bloody scene of the birth. Unconscious anxieties seem to relate to a primal scene exposure – witnessing a primitive scene of unpredictable, powerful passions from which he is physically excluded while emotionally involved. Male survivors of childhood abuse and family violence are especially prone to anxieties at this unleashing of primitive physical forces, and their own helplessness in the face of pain. If their trepidation remains undisclosed, expectant fathers find even videos of the birth shown in some preparation classes disturbing rather than reassuring. Unvoiced fantasies proliferate, and when attendance at the birth is foisted on him, physical fainting or practical sabotage may take over to protect the man from having to live out the highly arousing aspects of his birth sentence.

A prompt referral for psychotherapy may enable a man or couple to work through some of these feelings before the birth. When these are unavailable, frank communication in childbirth preparation classes and discussion of expectations and hesitations before the event may forestall bitter disappointments. A couple on the verge of splitting up talk in my consulting room about the events of the previous year, for the first time since the premature birth of their only child.

'What I can't forgive,' says the woman vehemently, 'is that he tricked me into believing he'd be at the birth, but when I found labour had started and I called to ask him to come, he delayed until it was all over.'

'I was working', he replies sullenly.

'But I needed you', she says plaintively. 'Our baby was getting born and you missed it.'

'I was there afterwards, and I did put up curtains in the baby's room while you were in hospital', he reminded her.

'That's easy stuff. I wanted you there to want to share the most important happening of our joint life, but you weren't there . . . You grow a lot when you're in touch with another person', she adds in an aside to me. 'When two people start sharing their lives, something happens to make you feel you trust the other to know your needs. I was beginning to feel that with him when I found I was pregnant. Not a great romantic ideal, but trust. That's what got killed while I lay there watching out for him and crying, wanting him there and waiting for him. I held on and held on, for hours – lost all sense of time – then something just caved in and I gave up on him, stopped holding it in and gave birth within minutes. When he sailed through the door of the ward, it was too late. I had lost too much. We can't ever go back there again.'

'You never told me how much it meant to you', he sobs.

'I suppose I was too frightened to know.'

'I don't think we've ever really spoken until now', she says sadly. 'And now there's nothing left to say . . .'

5
A Model of Differing Orientations

In an airy carpeted room, seven pregnant women sprawl as they talk about their feelings:

'This pregnancy business is certainly over-rated', says Lisa, fanning herself.

'I love being pregnant', Vicky croons. 'It makes me feel so special. I wish it could go on forever . . .'

'I'm enjoying this pregnancy,' says Maggie, 'but last time I couldn't stand the feeling of being both me and about to be taken over. I'd wanted a baby but hadn't bargained on enormous changes and no control. It was quite a relief when I miscarried at eleven weeks.'

'Last time my baby was late', Clarissa says, holding her very large bulge. 'It was as though my whole body clenched, not letting him go. I felt it was all so lovely, we were so close, and it wasn't safe to let him out. But once he *was* out we were close in a different way – I just devoted myself to his every wish. It's funny. This time, since twenty-eight weeks I've wanted pregnancy to be over. Sometimes I wish this baby could take care of itself, so I could go back to work and get on with my life.'

There is a brief silence. Then Shama adds thoughtfully, 'With my first, I was so shaken up by having a small thing so dependent on me that I escaped back to work after a few weeks. This time I know what to expect. I feel I have more to offer and won't be so afraid of being taken over. I'm already much more involved and quite looking forward to getting to know my baby.'

'Well, I'm not!' retorts Lisa emphatically. 'In the middle three months I had more energy. I used it as a lever to resign my job, but since I left work it's been terrible – I'm already so bored on my own that the prospect of staying home with a baby is horrific!'

'I'm not bored – or alone', remarks Esther, stroking her round tummy. 'I talk to my baby all the time, and what's more, she answers back.'

'Come off it! It's only a fetus, for goodness sake!' Lisa retorts scathingly.

'That's what people said when I had my miscarriage', Colleen says softly. 'But it was a baby I lost.'

There are as many responses to pregnancy as there are pregnant women. Some blossom and feel enriched; others fade and feel depleted. Some women give in to the emotional processes of pregnancy; others hold out against introspection. Some change their lifestyles to accommodate the pregnancy, others continue as before. As we saw in relation to the placental paradigm, some experience the baby as a benign presence, others treat it as a parasitic invader. Due to individual variations, emotional fluctuations over the course of pregnancy, and the uniqueness of each woman's internal world configurations, generalized descriptions of women – pregnant or otherwise – overlook crucial differences between them. It is thus important to bear in mind *the extraordinary variability of responses to pregnancy*. At the same time, however, I find it is possible to discern certain trends that may make sense of seemingly contradictory approaches to pregnancy, birth, and motherhood.

Divided into subgroups, research respondents reveal patterns which are swamped by treating the sample as a homogeneous group. Expectant mothers too sometimes find it useful to be described in a way which gives a unifying meaning to seemingly disparate factors, and increases their understanding of unconscious issues.

I've tried to find a way of clustering tendencies in mothering that begin during pregnancy and persist across the child's developmental phases, in a model flexible enough to respond to changes in the mother's emotional and socio-economic conditions, including the birth of subsequent children. I've also sought to construct a model which could operate cross-culturally, yet take account of local childrearing practices. Although far from ideal, these categories are not diagnostic, judgemental nor intended to conjure up stereotypes, but rather delineate several common styles of response and the beliefs underpinning them.

In reality few people are pure types, and the picture presented is a composite of many different women.

Over the last decade, the model has undergone elaboration as my understanding has increased. This presentation therefore is more complex. Originally composed of a continuum between two points – Facilitators and Regulators – I have come to recognize that the model is not linear but circular, with the intermediary group having a philosophy and identity of their own, as Reciprocators. Recent studies suggest a necessity to include a fourth, 'bipolar' category, of conflicted people who embrace both extreme positions at once.

The Facilitator

'I feel very turned on and tuned in all the time, and want everybody to know I'm pregnant, even though it doesn't show yet. I feel round and abundant and wonder-full.'

A woman of the first orientation usually becomes aware of conception very early on. With a frisson of excitement, she feels she is no longer alone but contains a *secret* ticking away within her. Immediately on assuming she is pregnant, she gives herself over to the heightened emotionality of pregnancy, steering clear of situations and substances she fears may be harmful, changing her diet and habits. She aims to devote herself to facilitating the baby's wellbeing – prenatally, postnatally, or even through preconceptual care. Excitedly sharing her news, she carefully examines the responses of her confidantes, wishing them to be as thrilled and as proud of her marvellous achievement as she feels of herself. Experiencing pregnancy as the culmination of her feminine identity, she feels privileged by comparison to her male partner, who has only indirect access to the baby.

Transformed by her new state, which grants fulfilment of a long-postponed childhood wish, she feels herself becoming an active link in the chain of pregnant females since time immemorial, joining her mother, born of *her* mother, and *her* mother before. The newly pregnant Facilitator thus becomes caught in a series of interchangeable identifications, feeling merged with both she who carried her, and with the baby now residing inside her womb – as she herself was carried within her mother's body.

Over the next weeks, as her conception assumes permanence, the Facilitator begins to rejoice in symptoms such as nausea and nipple pigmentation, which reinforce her confidence in the reality of her invisible pregnancy. 'I so want to get bigger,' says Vicky in her ninth week, 'so that what I feel inside myself can actually be seen, and other people will believe it.' Indeed, she may feel tempted to begin wearing maternity clothes before the 'bump' even begins to show. Social contacts may become restricted to a select circle of intimates as her centre of gravity shifts inwards, and she feels absorbed in thoughts about the magical process taking place within her.

The Regulator

'I've not allowed myself to change,' says mother-to-be Sabrina in an in-depth interview. 'I've seen a lot of women lose their identities and become boring. I haven't changed my routine nor my clothes much, and didn't tell anyone I was pregnant. I think many women just use pregnancy as an excuse to be lazy and self-indulgent, and to gain extra attention: "Look at me! Look at me!" '

At the other end of the spectrum we find the woman who wishes to regulate her life. To her, pregnancy is a rather tedious means of getting a baby. Tending to avoid the pull towards introspection, which she regards as a sentimental indulgence, she also decides not to share her news with anyone outside her immediate intimates until she is well and truly pregnant. Unlike the Facilitator, who relishes the special treatment accorded pregnant women, the Regulator may insist on being treated as usual, finding it quite insulting to be addressed as if she were a pregnancy – or indeed a Regulator – rather than herself. Finding the reappraisal of identity foisted on her by pregnancy quite disconcerting, she resolves to minimize changes to her lifestyle and internal world, establishing herself as autonomous and detached. Despite tiredness she may actually step up her social life, determined not to be taken over by her symptoms. She is prepared to let the 'bump' tag along, but not to let it become the focus of her being.

The Reciprocator

'It's hard to go on with work and the rest of my life acting as if there's no change', says a pregnant mother of three teenagers. 'I need recuperation time from tiredness and discomfort, but I also need time to consolidate my career before the birth. Although I love being with my family, I want to be on my own, to relish this pregnancy, which I know will be my last.'

Aware from the start of her ambivalence, a female Reciprocator is both overjoyed to be pregnant, yet regretful too of inevitable changes that are bound to occur in her own professional and personal life, and as a family or childless couple. While excited at the prospect, in becoming parents, Reciprocators are rare in being able to anticipate realistically the changes this may entail in their relationship as lovers, free agents, and helpmates. While the pregnancy does not dominate their lives, it adds a new richness and warmth to the couple's experience of each other as potential parents to a baby of their making: 'Part of the fun of having kids is finding out what the mix of your genes makes.'

The expectant Reciprocator with no steady partner may have chosen to become pregnant and gone to some lengths to do so. Or if her pregnancy is unplanned, after some deliberation she might have made an informed choice in keeping it, knowing of her own ambivalence, aware of both joyful and difficult times ahead:

'I know it won't be easy bringing up a child alone, but I'm thirty-seven and time is running out. I've always wanted a child, and couldn't just leave it to fate. If in the future I meet someone I can spend the rest of my life with, that will be wonderful. Meanwhile, I'll do the best I can with help from my family and friends.'

In the first trimester, although her whole life is coloured by the knowledge of her pregnancy, a Reciprocator tries to maintain a balance between inner absorption and an acute awareness of the world outside, in which she lives, works and will bring up her child. The hallmark of this orientation is a capacity to remain aware of ambivalence and internal contradictions.

These three orientations are not fixed personality characteristics, but are based on the current state of the mother's intrapsychic reality. Orientations may, and often do, change with a subsequent pregnancy:

'I'm already so aware of the baby as an individual – a future person to whom I will be introduced', says Sonia in the early weeks of pregnancy. 'With my little girl, Sophie, I couldn't visualize her at all during pregnancy except as a miniature version of myself, and when she was born I devoted myself to giving her everything I would have loved to have had as a baby. I had no idea how she would develop into herself, or even that she would! But with this pregnancy, I realize the baby will be very much his or her own person, neither like me nor even like Sophie. But at the same time, because of my experience, I can imagine the new baby all the way up to her current age.'

Middle and Late Pregnancy

The Facilitator

For the Facilitator, once movement is experienced, the fetus who has up to now felt like part of her is recognized as a separate being albeit, as Sonia illustrates above, one who is unconsciously still part of the mother's self. Basking in the glow of pregnant potential, she reluctantly begins to differentiate herself from her baby and from her own mother. Simultaneously she spins fantasies about all the possible babies this one might be. Like a child in communion with an imaginary friend, she is never alone. She revels in the emotional tug, feeling enriched by an internal presence that only she can experience. It seems to her that other people treat her with a slight sense of awe, as if she has become greater than the sum of herself. Indeed, on an unconscious level she is finally full of herself, as idealized mother–baby facets of her internal world acquire substance with her swelling bulk.

Extreme Facilitators may resort to idealization as a defence against unmitigated unconscious hostility and destructiveness. Warding off any hint of ambivalence, a precarious internal state of bountiful bliss is maintained by externalizing the enemy, which may result in phobic fears of contamination, radiation, heights, flying, and water, or paranoid anxieties of assault or medical malpractice. In women with a psychosomatic tendency, bad feelings may be hived off into an organ or limb, which can both express and keep them imprisoned to protect the fetus.

In some cases, pregnancy may have been sought to serve narcissistic gratification, magically to close an internal rupture in a woman's profound failure to separate from her mother; or as an attempt to deny guilt and past regrets; or omnipotently to overcome anxieties inherent in ageing. If something goes wrong during the pregnancy or birth, this Facilitator may feel flooded with guilt or a sense of it all being 'spoilt' before it was even begun. When the fetus is deemed to reincarnate a lost loved one, or used to promote an omnipotent state of possessing both sexes within one body, the reality of birth and the baby are increasingly denied, until its inexorable imminence may impel the woman into a panic state or psychotic breakdown.

As we shall see in Chapters 10 and 11 psychodynamic treatment can enable a troubled woman to become aware of the unconscious emotional significance of her defences, and help her towards acceptance of her own ambivalence through lessening the repression of bad and hateful aspects of the self identified with internal persecutory figures.

The Regulator

The Regulator may feel at times as if she has been taken over by an invader, sapping her internal resources. Once movement is experienced, this feeling is exacerbated by the sense of something operating within her that remains beyond her control. She may resolve to protect herself from the intruder by looking after her body and replenishing her lost energy through special meals or extra naps. By stepping up social activities, and postponing 'coming out' in maternity gear, she may try to reinforce her identity as an independent, sexual woman, resenting her partner, who can have their baby without symptoms, disclosure and physical change.

Reluctant to invest the fetus with human personality traits, she forgoes fantasy and imaginary conversations with the fetus; many Regulators are amazed by pregnant Facilitators' unselfconscious 'prattling' to the baby. The Regulator justifies her stance as sensible, trying to maintain a familiar identity and sense of separateness in case something goes wrong.

Extreme Regulators may employ defensive techniques which enable them to remain unaware of primitive emotional states.

Anxieties may originate in a fear of exploitation and engulfment, or a sense of persecutory attack from the uncontrollable fetus, which is seemingly in cahoots with a bad internal figure; or there may be fears of her own badness and hostility damaging the fetus. Unlike the Facilitator for whom dangers lurk outside, a Regulator may have a sense of an enemy within. Defensive measures may involve schizoid splitting, dissociation or use of compulsive behaviour and rituals to hold obsessional conflicts at bay. The approaching birth exacerbates anxieties about inner damage and tearing, caused by a baby who is desperate to get out, and/or by unleashing of her own unrestrained aggressive urges.

By late pregnancy, feeling drained and ungainly, most Regulators are fed up with the internal battering and distracting kicking which affects both sleep and work. Some respond by intensifying detachment. Although eager to rid herself of her internal persecutor, the expectant mother may nevertheless be apprehensive about the ordeal of labour, resolving this dilemma by learning as much as possible about pain-reduction techniques and labour control.

'It's a very strange feeling – having something alien moving inside,' says Sabrina who we met above in early pregnancy. 'At first I felt invaded by this eavesdropping creature, listening in to every word I said and exploiting me, rotting my teeth and draining my energy. Now (eight months) that I've been given a crib and some clothes, it's beginning to be real, I'm making the connection that what's in here will go into this tiny vest. . . . People keep saying: "have you done . . . ? Have you bought . . . ?" but I wont do it yet, I can always order and have them delivered when the baby arrives. The main hurdle now is the labour. [. . .] I'm not one of those women who want to squat on the floor; I don't want a caesarean because of the scar and I'm put off an epidural because I can't endure the thought of a forceps delivery – those horrible big metal things – so I'll just have drugs and after it's born, well they can go and weigh it and then they give it to you, don't they or do they hang on to it? I don't know, I suppose it depends . . . I think I'd like them to bring it to me cleaned up. Maybe I'll just say, "God I'm so exhausted, give it to me when I wake up." Only thing is they might get them muddled up in the nursery. But I shall put myself in their hands and probably stay in there as long as I can.'

The Reciprocator

While she enjoys her pregnancy as a preparatory time, the Reciprocator is keen to have it end so she can meet the child she is carrying:

> 'I think about the baby a lot of the time', says a musician in her sixth month of pregnancy. 'I feel more plugged in, full of energy, and my thought processes are bound up with the baby so I seem rather vague to other people, not a separate individual – but the me people relate to is the pregnant me. I'm very happy looking forward to getting to know this baby. I don't feel anxious, although I worry about sleepness nights and my capacity to mother.
>
> 'As to the pregnancy – it's a welcome being inside, and I feel happy it's there. I invited it to be there – I feel it has taken over creatively, not invasively. The baby doesn't demand of me in a way which is unreasonable – it's a benevolent feeling. I become increasingly bound up with this creature moving around, and also observe him responding to things – like certain pieces of music. But I don't want to fantasize to the point of disappointment: this baby is a person with his or her own responses and a personality which I'm genuinely curious about. I don't want to inject my personal expectations – I'd rather wait and watch and get to know as these qualities unfold over a period of time. As to the birth, it will just take place, and I'll do what I can at the time.'

The Expectant Partner

In most societies, both baby girls and boys are nurtured primarily by women. One consequence of this is that for boys as well as girls primary identification occurs with a female rather than male figure. In cultures where there is a high premium on autonomy, the little boy's masculinity comes about through secondary identification with his father or a male figure. The early time under the female wing is negated by complete or partial 'dis-identification', to use Ralph Greenson's felicitous term, from the caregiving mother, who has become synonymous with infantile dependency. Depending on the strength of maternal and paternal vectors in their particular family constellation, and the degree of machismo in the subculture, some boys retain their nurturant qualities, whereas others disavow them, along with all things 'feminine'.

The Participator

An expectant father of this orientation wishes to participate as fully as he can in the pregnancy, birth, and primary child care. He has free access within himself to identification with the baby-growing, nurturing mother of his early childhood, and is capable of being tender and gentle without self-consciousness. Amazed by the miracle of pregnancy, he wishes he too could experience it. If he can trust his partner's capacity to grow a baby, he will contribute his share by caressing and talking to the baby in her belly, feeding it with love and semen, and looking after the woman carrying their child.

However, if his envy of the woman's capacity to bear a child gets in the way, he may be unable to tolerate her good experience, feeling compelled to spoil it or take it over. Friends may be regaled with his descriptions of her symptoms or of the ultrasound images, as if she was not there. He may become over-anxious about her work and eating habits, insisting on attending antenatal clinics to check on her progress and control her gestation of his child.

For some Participators, preoccupation with the archaic mother of infancy may lead to identification not with the pregnant woman, but with the fetus he once was. As his early feelings are reactivated, he may sometimes feel as helplessly dependent as the baby: for example, wanting to be looked after, or literally becoming impotent. Over-identification with the vulnerable fetus trapped inside may result in him seeing himself as the baby's spokesman, interpreting every ripple, and voicing the fetus's imagined thoughts and preferences. Faced with the basic fact of male exclusion from pregnancy, how the Participator has resolved his early feminine identifications will determine whether he can sublimate his maternal aspects into supporting his pregnant partner, or whether his envy and competitiveness propels him into rivalry, couvade or inseparability from the fetus.

The Renouncer

A man of this orientation is also acutely aware of the male/female divide of pregnancy. However, in his case, as early identifications with his pre-Oedipal female mother threaten to assert themselves, he may intensify his masculine attributes, and identification with his father and the traditional paternal role: 'Isn't it a big baby I put in there!' He finds it difficult to empathize with the woman's internal experiences, regards her moodiness and introspection with some alarm, and treats the antenatal clinic as woman's business. Nevertheless, he is concerned with the well-being of both his wife and child, and, if willing to attend, may find the experience of seeing the baby on ultrasound gives an exciting reality to the newcomer in his life.

Although it is difficult for a first-time father to imagine life with a baby, he may indulge in daydreams about teaching an older child, or playing games with his verbal son or daughter. Like most fathers, a Renouncer often wonders what kind of parents both he and his partner will become. Anxiety may be rooted in childhood memories of the kind of contact he had with his own parents, or fear of changes in their marital relationship once the baby arrives. Further anxiety may stem from inability to tolerate infantile neediness and mess.

The Reciprocator

A father-to-be of this orientation is well aware of having mixed feelings about his partner's pregnancy, the birth, and the baby. While similar to his woman in many respects, at this point in time their biological differences are very apparent. Although pregnancy may be regarded as a desirable state, it is also a source of discomfort for the woman, and he regrets leaving her to carry the burdens of pregnancy and pain of birth to produce their child. He is nevertheless aware of the pleasant experiences she is having, which he can only feel vicariously. Trying to cast himself back, he ponders how he felt when he was little, and what his baby might be experiencing now, inside the womb, and later, during the labour, birth, and in contact with the world.

It is this experience of continuity and simultaneity of different senses of his self, and the capacity to move imaginatively among them – young and old, masculine and feminine, big and little, good and bad – that helps Reciprocators to tolerate the ambiguity and ambivalence of their situation. This is often accompanied by self-reflectivity, an ability to think about the meanings of his thoughts and actions and their effects on others. In many ways, these characteristics make life more difficult, as the

Reciprocator of either sex has to bear lack of certitude. However, in major life events like childbearing, when it is often impossible to make predictions with certainty, the Reciprocator has the advantage of a flexible approach, and access to a variety of inner resources to call upon if the unexpected happens.

6
Changing Relationships

'Up to now, professionally, I am who I am because of what I do', says Gabriella, a highly placed professional woman in her early thirties. 'At present what I'm doing is being pregnant. Sometimes I'm so exhausted it's the only thing I can do with any vigour, concentrating on trying to keep this pregnancy going. It's so perturbing to think that I'm going to suddenly change into being a mother and be at home cut off from outside and dependent on my husband for news of the world. Everything is changing – my relationship to him, to my parents, to my body, to my women friends, my male colleagues, my work – it's no wonder my dream life is in turmoil. I seem to spend my nights trying to sort it all out.'

Partners

Of all chosen relationships, the intimate one between adult lovers is perhaps the most complex, offering a sanctuary for the intense interplay of multiple conscious and unconscious exchanges. For many couples, it is the closest equivalent to the primary emotional relationship with their own parents during childhood. Often partners are selected with uncanny precision to replicate loved or hated aspects of a parent, or to duplicate, validate, or mirror unexpressed or cherished selves. Emotional collusions occur in all close relationships, as receptive partners are unconsciously induced to enact scenes from their internal worlds. As I have suggested elsewhere, when the scenario is predetermined, as it is between partners who feed off each other, they may come to inhabit each other's fantasy worlds, rather than meeting as individuals in their own right.

In the transition to parenthood, pregnancy alters existing interactional patterns, precipitating change and offering opportunities to renegotiate emotional expectations. Even while looking forward to their first baby the expectant couple will inevitably experience concerns about having to share their intimate duo and emotional resources with a third. Oedipal anxieties are revitalized as a twosome turns into a triangle, and issues of possessiveness and rivalry come to the fore, as they did in child-hood conflicts. Twinges of jealousy and competitiveness, or anx-iety over loss of one's partner's full attention are common and inevitable. However, intense preoccupations with the triangular constellation often signify unresolved issues of inclusion/exclusion from the childhood parental couple.

Reciprocity between the partners is affected by pregnancy de-stabilizing the gender balance. Polarization of male-female dif-ferences may give rise to sexual problems, and redefine or exacerbate power and control dimensions in the partnership. Subsequent pregnancies too may reactivate seemingly resolved conflicts or arouse an unexplored range of feelings and the po-tential for new growth:

> 'It's taken me a long time to really look my partner in the eye at close quarters', says a pregnant woman, whose first child's conception almost coincided with the beginning of her rela-tionship. 'I keep being surprised by him. As if it's only during this pregnancy have I allowed him to become real in my mind. I suppose with one baby you can still think of splitting up, but with two it's a real family and you're all entwined. I thought I'd feel trapped, but it's actually brought us closer, made us communicate our feelings more now we're truly committed.'

Among heterosexual couples, even those who have confi-dently enjoyed an equal distribution of 'shares', pregnancy inev-itably emphasizes asymmetry. These differences become increasingly apparent for Gabriella, especially since she and her partner share the same profession:

> 'There is a new closeness between us', says Gabriella (a Re-ciprocator), in her eighth week of pregnancy. 'He's so happy it's palpable. At first he tried to be sensible to protect me from possible disappointment, but now it's secure, he's openly delighted – he keeps saying, "I'm going to be a father." At the same time, there is a separateness – this spe-cial experience denied to men, the sense of growing some-thing. He thinks I should be able to pull out of it like he switches off at work. But I can't; it's always there. It's worst in the evenings when I'm forced inward by tiredness and feeling sick. I find we're having two separate conversations

about our day, not a dialogue. We really have to make an effort to hear each other . . .'

Although individual responses vary a great deal, and change at different times during the pregnancy, as unconscious forces take over, the bedrock of biological fact and bodily experience forces men and women to re-examine themselves as 'masculine' or 'feminine' – sometimes with unanticipated consequences. A determinedly independent woman may surprise herself by wanting to be pampered by her partner during pregnancy, or mothered by her mother or female friends. A woman who has been dependent or unassertive may experience a new freedom having achieved pregnancy; or she may feel she has found an internal companion, witness, or audience for her activities in the world. An empty woman may feel fuller and never alone; a full man may feel emptier and excluded.

'Jacob hardly figures at the moment.' Gabriella, fourteen weeks pregnant, lolls comfortably on the couch holding her bump. 'I do feel sorry for him. It's extraordinary to be able to grow a baby, a most peculiar phenomenon. My libido has just gone. In the first weeks we were worried because of spotting. Now I just want to go to sleep and dream my strange dreams. He's very patient, but must be fed up and feel excluded. I'm so sexually disinterested, and can't convey how I'm feeling. I'm sure sex would establish "us" again and renew our closeness, but I feel separate because I'm wrapped up in what is going on inside my body. I think I'm retreating from what could be an intrusion into the specialness of the baby and me . . . It's peculiar, I look the same but there's a baby growing contentedly inside me. There are two of us not one of me.'

As the momentum of the transition to parenthood gathers force, both partners may find work and intellectual preoccupations recede in their desire to find out more about babies. However, as Garbriella makes clear, he can forget 'they' are pregnant: she lives every moment of her waking life with the physical reality of it.

There are ways in which the pregnant woman and her mate, if she has one, may utilize the slow-motion impetus of awaiting the birth of their baby to become closer. This may include increasing their empathic responsiveness and mutual understanding by talking through fears and fantasies, and trying to comprehend what the other is feeling.

'This pregnancy has undoubtedly enriched our relationship', says Gabriella in her last weeks, feeling about to "pop". 'We've become more insular. At first this was imposed by my symptoms of nausea and tiredness, but also because we enjoy each other's company, despite the fact our sex life is again non-existent.

I've grown to love this child over the months, as if there's a peaceful centre inside me and in our home, whatever chaotic turmoil is going on in the rest of our lives and at work. In some ways I'm going to miss this lovely feeling of intimacy with the baby – it's the closest you can get to someone – but it will be nice to have a two-sided relationship, and birth will equalize our contact with the baby once it's outside. At the moment, my husband talks to me and I tell the baby what he's told me to say, as if he can't communicate with it directly. It will still be unequal while I'm feeding and at home, but we'll both enjoy finding out who this child is and what we're like as parents.'

During early pregnancy, a couple often draw in, becoming more home-centred and self-engrossed, in order to meet emotional and physical needs. There may be a realignment of relationships, as first-time parents gravitate towards friends who have greater expertise in pregnancy and parenting. Single friends and those who are involuntarily childless may be avoided out of a fear of being envied, particularly if the expectant couple have themselves been subfertile.

On the other hand, the need to talk about the process going on inside her pregnant body creates new bonds with other pregnant women, equally excited by the sense of joining the club of initiated mothers. The sense of sharing mysteries with female peers is reminiscent of the young teenager's identification with her community of girlfriends, who share the discovery of sexuality, menstruation, and girlish secrets.

The Daughter's Mother

'I got into a blind panic after telling my parents', says Gabriella early on. 'It felt like tempting fate. I was completely terrorized, as though I'd spoken out of turn and could arouse the "evil eye". It's bizarre how superstitious I've become . . .'

Throughout pregnancy, archaic feelings are triggered by unavoidable parallels between the mother-to-be holding a baby in her womb, and having been held in the womb of her own mother. What is reactivated is the ambivalence embedded in their gender similarity and primary bodily identification, which the male child does not share with his mother. This Russian-doll imagery of mothers and daughters one inside the other rekindles early anxieties and unresolved issues of love and hate between the pregnant woman and her internal mother (rather than the real one, who may or may not be alive).

A numinous network of intertwining impressions and fragmented memories rise from the depths of a woman's unconscious during pregnancy. These range from jubilant rapture to poignant tenderness, punctured by moments of frustration, anguish, loss, and betrayal and include her mother's old throwaway lines:

'You tore me up'; 'You smelled so good'; 'It was so excruciating'; 'I never regained my figure'; 'Your birth was easier than your brother's.' 'I had to have my varicose veins stripped after you'; 'I loved breastfeeding'; 'Feeding made my breasts sag'; 'Look at those stretchmarks'; 'Pregnancy is a lovely period'; 'Never again'. . .

Like all relationships, the mother-daughter one is marked by a mixture of feelings. Here, however, the origins are deeper, stretching back to the womb. Even a woman who had been overjoyed by conception may suddenly feel irrationally furious at the thought of her baby receiving the tender loving care of which she herself feels deprived. Early battles rage within her, as old jealousies, hurts, and anxieties flare up in all their potency:

'Yesterday I had tears streaming down my face as I recalled how I pinched and tormented my baby brother when mother brought him home from hospital', says Miriam who referred herself for treatment during pregnancy because of severe panic attacks. 'My period would have been due, and I got scared, feeling I was sure to miscarry. In my head I could hear my mother's voice saying: "Did you really think you could get away with it?" I felt doomed to lose my baby as punishment for persecuting hers.'

Women who cannot come to grips with the inevitability of their mixed feelings may be stuck with a rigidly guarded, split, and unrealistic image of the mother. This will be expressed in an over-idealized mother who is omnipotently perfect and therefore an unobtainable model for mothering. Alternatively, the internal mother will seem to be a sinister and powerfully controlling, malevolent presence or an elusive, indefinable one. There may then be the need to protect herself from real or imagined maternal rivalry or hostility. Such a woman may have to go to great lengths to define herself as separate and different from the powerful maternal image she carries about inside. A not infrequent solution consists of disavowing the 'witch' and ascribing some of the mother's positive attributes to another, older woman – sometimes a health care professional – who can then act as mother figure, and provide some of the maternal care that many pregnant women yearn for.

Trying to be 'good', an emotionally dependent woman might feel tempted to hand over her antenatal care, birth, and baby to her mother, who has always done it all for her: 'If my mother's there, she'll make it all right.' A woman who has remained in a fused, cloying relationship with her possessive or reciprocally dependent mother may also contrive to give the baby to her mother to look after, or to be shared within their circle of intimacy. The newborn may symbolize her reincarnated baby self, or the fantasy baby she and mother have mutually brought into being: 'I was my mother's whole life; the baby let us re-live it', said Sonia about baby Sophie.

A more self-reflective woman might grasp this belated opportunity to struggle out of her bondage by contriving to make pregnancy a private experience: 'I just pretend I'm not in when she calls.' Asserting disputed rights over her body by flaunting her emotional autonomy, a woman may refuse advice or help and sometimes go to foolhardy lengths to establish her emancipation, even repeatedly conceiving and aborting in unconscious insubordination. Another may express her internal conflict by setting herself up to be the 'opposite' to her mother: 'She must have spent her entire pregnancy complaining. You won't hear a peep out of me.'

With the superstitious logic of the irrational, a woman whose own mother had miscarriages, obstetric complications, a stillbirth, or handicapped baby may feel particularly vulnerable during her pregnancy, finding it difficult to believe she will be allowed to have a creative experience without feeling guiltily triumphant, or anxious about retaliation: 'My mother had a Caesarean section for her first child. I can't believe I'll get away with a normal birth. My sister did, so maybe I'll have to pay.'

Unless the complex, unconscious issues underlying such behaviours are emotionally worked through and outgrown, merely excising the mother does not prevent a woman from repeating the same overbearing intimacy with her child and/or partner. On the contrary, the call from the deep reasserts itself as a craving for emotional merger or determined immunity to it, manifest in over-involved maternal exclusivity, or its reverse.

Daughters who in adolescence rebelliously resisted identification with their mothers and have achieved their own individuation may now feel free to utilize pregnancy to ratify their femininity. A new compassion may arise born of the shared female experience. Other women may find the conflictual mother-daughter relationship persists, and is in fact aggravated by their pregnant vulnerability.

Given readiness for change, and the impetus of becoming a mother herself, pregnancy offers a fine opportunity for women who feel they have unresolved internal struggles with their mothers to explore these with therapeutic help. As Miriam, who was quoted above, says in the last trimester of her pregnancy:

'There's a dawning realization that an ideal mother isn't going to emerge out of mine. Somewhere along the line, I set up this paragon mother and have been so engrossed in what it could be like if only she would change that I haven't really recognized what is actually there, on offer.'

The Parents' Parents

Pregnancy heightens awareness of connections between the generations, highlighting emotional correspondences and differences in the expectant parent's relationship to her or his parents, dead or alive. In adopted mothers-to-be, divided loyalties and old conflicts often resurface as a woman is torn between identifying with the woman who carried but relinquished her, and the care-providing, adopting parents who now await their grandchild. Conception may have come in the wake of a parental loss, or as a reparatory gift to an unhappy parent, unconsciously hoping to boost an ailing mother or father, or to fill a gap in their lives.

Even with a planned pregnancy, old prohibitions on sexuality, or unconscious rivalries may re-emerge. Telling may also evoke primitive fears of not being allowed to keep the baby. Feeling anxious about her disclosure, which looms with disapproval, a woman may put off telling her parents that she is expecting a child. Their reaction takes on extreme importance as a reflection of their response to the news of her own arrival:

> 'I'm dying to call my parents, but know I may be sorely disappointed. I want them to be thrilled and feel I've done something great. I want them to be happy and proud. But my mother has never learned to respond with an uncomplicated "Yippee!" Her response will be, "You're what?! Don't tell anyone until three months in case you miscarry"', says Daniel's mother in the first weeks of her second pregnancy.

In some families, a woman may feel uneasy about revealing her pregnancy, treating it, and/or being treated, as if the pregnancy was proof of disloyalty to her father or family of origin. In possessive families, even as a fetus, a baby may become a pawn in a power struggle between in-laws, as claims are staked and information about the pregnancy shared or witheld, and control is established over the expectant parents and their baby through advice or emotional blackmail.

While for some couples pregnancy reactivates childish anxieties, for others a first pregnancy may consolidate a new adult relationship with the parents – as if they had not really considered their daughter or son to be truly grown up until this time. Paradoxically, alongside this ratification of maturity there may be an enhanced recognition of being the parents' child. The expectant parents luxuriate in the sense of having satisfied *their* parents' wish to be grandparents, while the latter bestow solicitous care on the beloved daughter or son, who (temporarily) can do no wrong.

Women whose fathers have seemed aloof and distant may welcome pregnancy as a second chance to gain closeness:

'I'm afraid to tell my father. I have a fantasy my pregnancy will kill him off', says one of my patients on first discovering she is pregnant. Three weeks later she says: 'Since I told him I'm pregnant, my relationship with my father is easier. He's quite excited. I thought he'd be flat, but he really is very pleased for me – it's nice seeing him so enthusiastic. He told me he'd been frightened of having a baby, but he *was* glad I was born. Suddenly so much acrimony has just evaporated.'

The above vignette illustrates not only the superstitious connections between life and death, intuitive understanding, and healing powers of pregnancy, but how confirmation of an unconscious suspicion – in this case of the father's early trepidation – can ease unspoken tension of years' standing.

These wide-open potentialities of pregnancy as a second chance and new beginning incite the imagination of all those closely involved. Paradoxically, the shared experience of the generations – each mother having been a daughter, and each father having been a son – enables the older couple to relinquish their personal claims at the very moment of possessively establishing them. In most cases, in granting the younger their place in the chain of generations, the older couple will more or less generously step aside. In turn, as the mother- and father-to-be begin to contend with the everyday difficulties of becoming parents, gradually recognizing their own fallibility, they forgive that of their own caregivers.

Siblings

'I said to Daniel, "I've got a baby in my tummy." "No!", said he. Then, puffing out his jumper, he declared, "I've got one too!" Some days later, he put his lips right up to my abdomen and said "Baby – I'm so glad to meet you. Come on out." But later two-and-a-half-year-old Daniel said, "I want to get inside your tummy and squash the baby out of there." '

Obstetricians refer to pregnancies as unrelated events each of which can be viewed in isolation. However, psychologically, each conception is affected by all past conceptions, and will affect all future ones. Likewise, as reshuffling of the family constellation occurs, all members of a family will be affected. This often necessitates realignment of increasingly complex emotional interconnections. In sheer numbers, each new arrival creates many new relationships. In fact, the formula $n(n-1)$ charts the geometric progression so that a second child increases the interrelations from six to twelve, and a third child brings it to twenty, and so on.

Complex interactions between such factors as number and age gap between children, psychosocial circumstances, as well as the degree of practical, emotional, and economic support she receives affect a woman's capacity to respond favourably to the rest of the family during the pregnancy and after the birth. The mother of a small child will have to loosen the mental grasp of her older baby in order to make place for the new one – a transition that may only finally take place after the birth, or, in some cases, never. In addition to welcoming a stranger, young siblings will have to make difficult concessions, yielding territory, possessions, and some attention to the newcomer, while abdicating a precious place in the family hierarchy. During pregnancy the mother's psychic space becomes occupied with the baby growing within her. Her thoughts stray to the child she holds inside, even while she interacts with the child on her lap, who will often become aware of, and sometimes draw attention to, her emotional lapses. At other times she may be poignantly aware of the inevitable rent in their intimacy which the new baby will bring about, feeling aching tenderness towards her older child, to whom she more intensely devotes herself than before. As Daniel's mother says some weeks later:

> 'I'm in a peculiar frame of mind – I'm so attached to Daniel and afraid. Could I ever love another baby? It took me so long to really get to know him. And if it's a girl my feelings will be so complicated because of my relationship with my mother and sister. I'm not ready to meet the baby yet; this time with Dan is so precious.'

Following the birth, the older sibling is not only deprived of his or her mother's ordinary loving attention, now diverted to the baby, but also divested of extra emotional involvement. Three-year-old Daniel demonstrated this following his sister's birth. When someone suggested the baby had caught his cold, he complained, 'She can't have *my* cold! It's *mine*!'

Babies become entangled in emotional strands that originated long before their conception. They are born into a preconstructed network to occupy a specific emotional place in the family. Sometimes one child is singled out for special treatment: unconscious connections between this baby and birth order in the constellation of her own childhood family can interfere with a woman's spontaneous investment in the child as a person in his or her own right. The new baby may come to represent an envied, beloved, hated, or pitied older or younger brother or sister. The mother may find it difficult to relinquish her special intimacy with an older child, resenting the new baby's intrusion. She may relegate one child to the emotionally neglected position of second-best. The mother may feel she herself or one of her siblings was allocated this place in childhood, and thus takes revenge on the newcomer as if it was her own sibling: 'My wife treats the baby like her younger brother. She despises his weakness and almost taunts him with it, as if she loses sight of this tiny, helpless creature.' Her mother's favouritism or prejudice towards a sibling may be transferred to the baby or to another child. These sentiments may be unconsciously delegated to another family member, to be enacted on her behalf while she consciously 'opposes' them.

Work

The issue of work and childbearing affects women worldwide. In Western countries, postponement of childbearing to facilitate career building means that many would-be-mothers have a high degree of responsibility in their non-domestic jobs. For each woman the issue of returning to work involves personal dilemmas in balancing the desire for self-actualization with the demands of pregnancy and mothering according to her own orientation. Given a choice, many Regulators return to full-time employment, while Facilitators delay doing so during the first two years, and some Reciprocators go back to part-time work. Even in the case of women who elect to work rather than being compelled to, the stress of doing the job to their own high standards, without any concessions or acknowledgement of their difficulties, is a telling indictment of the system:

'Work places rarely make allowances for the physical and emotional exertion of being a parent', complains the mother of two young children, trying to continue her professional commitments part-time. 'Employers forget or block out what a struggle it is for the parent of a young child just to remain civilized at this juncture. While a baby is dependent or when a toddler is ill, we have to cut out all but the essentials in our lives. There is no longer place for niceties as we get down to basics. At times I arrive at the office leaking milk from breastfeeding at all hours of the night, almost disinhibited from disturbed sleep and chronic tiredness, and tense to breaking point – yet I have to behave with my colleagues as though I've just read the newspaper over a leisurely breakfast in a civilized home.'

The stress begins during pregnancy. Far from compensating for the very considerable physical discrepancies between female and male partners during childbearing, in most countries there are social restrictions that actually perpetuate the gender divide. Studies conducted in Europe reveal a high rate of sickness-absence from work during pregnancy, particularly in women whose jobs entail physical or psychological strain. My own case-load indicates that work patterns vary for different women at different stages of pregnancy, depending on how each expectant mother feels about the demands of her specific job and the meaning her work assumes at this time in her life. Implicated too are the dictates of her socio-economic situation, cultural expectations, and the explanatory beliefs in her society. I'll quote Gabriella again, since she and her husband share a high-powered profession:

'Although I'd always expected to take time off after the birth, I hadn't realized how much my work would be affected by my tiredness, nausea, and lack of concentration during pregnancy. Men aren't affected when they have babies, but I suppose they also lose out. When I'm treated at work as if I should tuck it away and take no notice of the pregnancy, my defiant retaliation is to feel special. And it's true – I *am* doing this amazing thing. It's also true that I'll be allowed maternity leave and to be with the baby while Jacob's not, although it's just as much a period of turmoil for him. But he gets excluded — at the most he'll get two weeks paternity leave. On the other hand, he treats his job hours as fixed, and I already know that I'll resent being the one who will have to rush back in time for the nanny. It's always the women who have to bend.'

In the first phase of pregnancy when many women are nauseous and feel extremely fatigued, jobs that make heavy physical demands – or repetitive work, even while seated – can feel depleting. Women vary in their responses to their work burdens: some try to get sick leave so they can rest, while others feel better if occupied and in the company of other people, rather than feeling sick on their own at home. Despite her need to slow down, a reticent woman may be reluctant to admit publicly that she is pregnant when requesting time off. Similarly, a woman working with hazardous substances or heavy equipment may experience a dilemma, particularly if she is superstitious or has decided to keep the news to herself until she is clear of the risk of miscarriage. Secrecy, however, has its own hazards:

'Although it's only six weeks, and I haven't even told my parents or best friends, I've had to tell the lab technicians since there are radio-isotopes and toxic chemicals involved in my work', says a biochemist. 'I also feel I must protect myself from emotional danger at work. The last time I was pregnant, I told nobody. I had a burst of energy and got very active, then when I miscarried nobody knew and I took no time off, except the day I was doubled up with pain. As a result I had no proper period of grief and mourning – no acknowledgement and no healing time, which just left me with a blur of shame and a sense of failure I've only recently overcome. If I were to lose it this time I realize it isn't selfish to say I need time to get over it; I think I could face it publicly, not as something shameful, but a sorrow that warrants sympathy and support.'

Most women feel fit and full of energy during the second phase. Conscious of time passing and the uncertainties ahead, this period is often used to consolidate previous productivity. Some women actually step up their work activity at this time; others resent having to concentrate on work rather than being allowed to focus on the lively fetus, and have time to luxuriate in being pregnant.

'My ideal pregnancy would be to spend the next months in some peaceful villa in Tuscany, just concentrating on the pregnancy and my baby, and sorting myself out', says Gabriella in mid-pregnancy. 'I don't want to stay home because I'll be missing out on the challenges of my work, but I can't just get on with an ordinary day's work and ignore my pregnancy either. That will be my anxiety afterwards too, when the child is growing up and I'll be feeling I'm working away, missing out on the once-ever chance to see milestones before the moment passes. It's a terrible conflict, because if I take a year off or put my career on a slow burner, I won't be able to go back to the fast lane – there are all these young guns coming up behind me, all happy to take that place.'

As the final phase approaches, some women crave the arrival of long-awaited maternity leave – others are filled with panic at replacing the familiar security of a working day with unstructured time. Comparing studies across Europe, in most countries all but twenty per cent of women stop work by thirty-two weeks. As always, internal factors may be found to interact with external ones, as the woman's relation to her job, to her partner, mother, baby, and beliefs about work, idleness, rest and entitlement each play their part:

'I tell myself I'm trying to establish my work as much as I can before going on leave,' says Miriam, who is self-employed, 'but inside my head it's as if I hear my mother's voice saying there should be no concessions for tiredness. I also feel terrified that once the baby comes I'll be incapacitated and unable to get back to the same workload. It's only in these last few weeks since the midwife gave me permission to do only what can't be avoided that I've slowed down. This coincided with the baby shifting downward onto my pubic bone. I was frantic that the head was being engaged, and that it would be six weeks early. The midwife told me to talk to the baby to tell it to stay inside for a few more weeks. I was so wiped out, I stayed in bed for a day and relaxed, and the baby seems to have shifted again.'

Knowing when to stop work is compounded for many women by a sense of failure in asking for special treatment, or even admitting to tiredness, as a doctor discovered:

'I'm shocked at myself. I've had this romanticized image of pregnancy, but it's quite hard work – a whole separate job, and I haven't had an uninterrupted night's sleep for months. It's unreasonable to think one can carry on a job regardless, but there's this strange sense of a split personality: me content to just feel my bump and commune with the baby, and my angst-ridden other self racing round like a blue-arsed fly, pressurized to clear the slate before the birth.'

Work expectations during pregnancy are an example of pressures on women to squeeze into inappropriate male standards. For some women, admission of their limitations may be a relief, breaking down the split maintained between polished professional and ordinary private personae. Discovering she is entitled to consideration anticipates the hard times ahead when the professional-woman-cum-mother inevitably will be less than perfectly prepared for her job, or will have to overcome internal reprimands to seek concessions because of trying to meet her baby's needs as well as those of her boss.

The Professional Woman

The particular nature of a woman's job is very significant. Professions involving a close, caring relationship with other people – like teaching, nursing, or counselling – are particularly taxing. This is not only because the woman is having to give from her own emotional resources, but, transferring feelings from their childhoods as she grows larger, her clients may be threatened by the power of her fertility and angry about her imminent maternity leave, causing her in turn to feel guilty, both for being pregnant and for leaving them. Punishing her and testing her endurance and devotion, they tend to impose extra demands on her patience.

Dependent clients, envious colleagues, and others who have found the birth of younger siblings traumatic often resent the professional's pregnancy to the point of making it the target of direct or concealed verbal attacks. She may then experience a compulsion to protect her baby and herself both physically and psychically by retreating inwards, and/or curtailing her work. It is particularly difficult if her job demands listening and giving the client her full attention, when she is distracted by the call of her own inner feelings and is trying to filter out communications she imagines could be disturbing to her fetus:

'I feel exhausted', says a concerned psychotherapist. 'It's taken all my resources to deal with an extremely envious woman without entering into the perverse script she was writing for me. I had to tell myself to be realistic – that I have a right to be pregnant; that although my patient desperately wants to be pregnant herself, I can't make her that; nor can I give up my own pregnancy for her. But it's hard to be generous and understanding while being on the receiving end of her envy and rage. With other patients, it's so difficult to take their punitiveness without wanting to retaliate or to empathize with inconsolable feelings, when I myself feel so vulnerable.' (See also Chapters 10 and 11.)

In other professions like law and medicine, women might feel enraged by the double standard that condones time out for research or study leave, but penalizes women who have taken maternity leave. Many professional women resent having to anticipate future arrangements before they have had the experience on which to base their decisions. Another source of resentment is the stark alternatives some careers pose: full-time work or ultimate demotion.

In addition to having to keep up with her peers, a working woman may be doubly disadvantaged, having to compete with men who have supportive wives while she has to fulfil domestic duties in addition to her job. When children enter the equation, unless she has access to domestic help and child care the struggle to maintain her career status may become too demanding. The personal and societal loss – not only of earnings and training but of ambition, solid experience, competence, and self-esteem – is immeasurable.

What is important is for each woman to understand her own orientation during pregnancy: only she can know her capacities and emotional priorities, or gauge her limitations. Many women learn during pregnancy to find ways of looking after themselves rather than being driven by unrealistically high standards, whether external or internal. Similarly, postnatally, some women are economically dependent on their income, or cannot afford to neglect their professional skills, or to break the momentum of their career. Others could take time off from work but choose not to out of a sense of achievement from, commitment to, or interest in, their work. A balance may be achieved by job sharing or flexible hours which allow a woman to replenish her adult 'stocks' and sense of public agency, while benefitting from the joys of parenting.

The difficulty in predicting her postnatal feelings across the Great Unknown complicates a pregnant woman's relationship to her work. In some countries this dilemma is eased by prolonged maternity leave with full pay, or at least a secure job that is held for her. This enables a new mother to make realistic choices based on actual experience with her particular baby, rather than hearsay, economic necessity, or fear of losing her job. Self-employed people and those in more flexible professions may have the freedom to postpone making decisions.

As unemployment rises, a natural experiment may take place, as many fathers too find themselves at home minding the baby, unable to determine the course of their own lives. Whereas primary care giver fathers who choose full-time parenting have been found to be most stimulating nurturers, when they have no choice will these reluctant first-time carers show the forbearance of countless generations of housebound mothers?

7
Conceived Realities – Technological Gains – and Loss

He laughed like an irresponsible foetus.
His laughter was submarine and profound
Like the old man of the sea's
Hidden under coral islands

T. S. Eliot, 'Mr. Apollinax'

Rethinking Preconceptions

In the West we are living through a time of extraordinary changes. Traditional extended families have been dismantled in favour of nuclear units. Rising life expectancy, coupled with safer childbearing and smaller families means Western women no longer spend most of their adult lives in a state of reproductive activity. Despite their shortcomings, female-controlled contraception and the sexual liberalization of women has enabled us to distinguish more clearly between sexuality, reproductivity, and female identity. It is now feasible to be feminine without being a mother; to become pregnant and choose not to have a baby; intercourse need no longer be associated with fear of conception. Today, when we not only can ensure sex without pregnancy, but pregnancy without sex, we are having to reformulate every aspect of our thinking about sexual differences, as even the foundations of the most elementary facts of life are being revised. Embryological research has come up with truth-stranger-than-fiction findings. It seems that before five weeks, irrespective of chromosomal markers, all embryos are essentially female until some are triggered hormonally to develop male characteristics.

With donor sperm and self-insemination, single mothers, and lesbian families, impregnation can occur without sex, or even a man. With *in vitro* fertilization and surrogacy, heredity can be ensured without pregnancy. New reproductive techniques, extending to ovum donation, mean a woman can carry a genetically unrelated baby, and gestation can override the time barrier of menopause. Technological advances in freezing embryos means that babies may be born of dead parents, or twins born years apart.

Although lagging behind somewhat, gradually societal norms come to reflect the choices behind these changes – sanctioning a woman's right to choose to not become a mother, to mother without a father, or even to be a mother without mothering. But do our internal worlds keep up with external changes? Having choices implies decision-making and acceptance of the consequences. It has become more difficult to be a parent now that social traditions and extended family structures and strictures are no longer available to guide us. The general shake-up of cultural attitudes to authority figures and invigorated sense of self-expression have resulted in a burgeoning of creative approaches to child care. This in turn means that the so-called experts are no longer granted the status they used to have. All parents can do is to make their own choices, driven by a desire to find a mode of mothering or fathering with which they feel most comfortable.

Luckily, babies have neither knowledge of 'ideal' parenting, nor do they arrive with preconceived notions about care. Being ordinary humans, they just want ordinary human care: understanding, recognition, acceptance, and loving contact. Evolution seems to have built the answer into the system: the very fact of having themselves been babies makes mothers and fathers potentially responsive if they can bear knowing that they, too, have been relatively needy, dependent and helpless and have experienced similarly intense feelings. Intuitive understanding is increased by a capacity to identify with human experience, whatever their sex. As the baby's raw feelings evoke the parent's psychic and sensory memories of that early time, depending on the quality of their own infantile emotional experiences, and the current climate of their internal worlds, those who can tolerate remaining receptive will respond sympathetically.

However, cultural valorization of independence and non-emotiveness, mean that to many parents it is precisely this capacity to arouse and bring about a return of the repressed, that makes babies dangerous (and addictive). And even though these registers remain unverbalized and may have long been suppressed, close contact with a baby thus activates a deep unconscious form of psychosomatic understanding. Some of these empathic feelings begin during pregnancy, as the parent tries to imagine what it must be like for the baby to be floating around in the womb like an astronaut tethered in space, receiving and transmitting bio-social 'messages', and rapidly growing bigger until there is only room for the occasional stretch within the confined watery balloon before eviction. With routine ultrasound screening, parental fantasy is supplemented by visualization of the somersaulting baby long before it arrives. No longer can the baby in the womb be imagined as an inactive blob.

'Belly-Button Window'

Innovatory procedures such as intrauterine photography, phonendoscopic recordings, and increasingly refined sonography have given us a glimpse of life inside the womb.

To my mind, one of the most extraordinary implications of fetal research discoveries of recent times is that *some capacities in the fetus greatly exceed those of newborns*. Indeed, some locomotor functions, like the ability to roll over, are not able to be used again until four or five months postnatally, so hampered is the infant by gravity.

Reviewing neonatal research findings, Chamberlaine concluded that by the second trimester of pregnancy, all human senses are operative. This indicates that the fetus is responsive to tactile, auditory, visual, kinaesthetic, vestibular (balance), gustatory (taste), thermic (heat and cold), and painful stimuli. The fetus is not only responsive, but assertive, both moving to increase his or her own comfort, and inducing changes in maternal physiology. As Liley states, he or she not only determines the length of the pregnancy and guarantees its endocrine success, but single handedly solves the problem of immunological incompatibility.

From around eight weeks, when movements are first observed on ultrasound, the fetus spends a great deal of time moving about. Many of these movements are never experienced by the mother, since sensation is conveyed not by the insensitive uterus, but by contact with the abdominal wall; in forty percent of pregnancies maternal sensation is cushioned by the location of the placenta on the front wall of the uterus. Ultrasound observations show how during the first half of pregnancy, lacking a gravitational axis of stability, the unrestricted fetus is capable of doing incredible somersaults and pirouettes. Such activity is now regarded as beneficial for the proper development of fetal muscles, bones, and joints.

Each fetus has his or her own cyclical patterns of daily activity, seemingly unrelated either to maternal activity or circadian rhythm. However, during the second half of pregnancy, the uterine space becomes progressively more ovid, and the growing fetus elongates more rapidly than the uterus. In this tapering, pear-shaped environment, the baby is increasingly restricted, and many movements are made in search of a more comfortable position, particularly once amniotic fluid volume begins to diminish after thirty-two weeks. The pre-labour Braxton-Hicks contractions of the uterine wall, the mother's perambulations, and her external palpations, all provoke the fetus to change position.

As the Italian psychoanalyst Alessandra Piontelli has demonstrated so graphically, ultrasound reveals that each fetus seems to develop favoured behavioural patterns which continue postnatally. She describes baby Guilia's prenatal tongue sucking or sensuous licking of the cord; Gianni hanging on to it like a rope or anchor while covering his face with his hands; and various twins, such as Marco using the placenta as a cushion for his head, and to protect him from his sister Delia's vigorous kicking.

Far from being passive, the fetus looks after his or her own needs. During the early period, if the budding hands accidentally touch the mouth, the embryo opens its lips but turns its head away. However, by twelve weeks the movement is reversed, and, like a newborn, the fetus turns towards the source of pressure, responds with sucking movements when the lips are touched, and may insert a thumb, finger, or toe into his or her mouth. In the fourth month, swallowing reflexes are activated as amniotic fluid is ingested and excreted in preparation for future digestion. Sometimes in later pregnancy mothers experience their baby's hiccups as a series of little rhythmic jolts. Experiments show that already in the early prenatal months babies feel pain and are discriminating: they jerk away from an intrusive needle, grimace at unpleasant tastes, and if sweet substances like saccharine are injected into the amniotic fluid, their swallowing rate doubles. Far from the placenta supplying all fetal needs, one theory is that by digesting the constituents of the amniotic fluid, calorie intake is increased, raising the possibility of fetal malnourishment being due to apathy!

That hearing is also discriminatory, expectant mothers have long known. Recordings made by a minute microphone inserted into the womb reveal that many ordinary external sounds are muffled by the internal whooshing of pulsating maternal blood flow and digestive noises. In addition, since the baby's eardrum is emersed in fluid on both sides, sounds are dampened, although higher frequencies suffer less loss than low ones in transmission through tissues and fluid. Thus the baby not only hears and startles to loud external noises, but listens to the mother's voice, and recognizes it postnatally, preferring his mother's voice over other women's, and even more remarkably, as DeCasper has shown, remembering it, and favouring stories read during pregnancy over new ones. Newborns also have been found to recognize, recall, and prefer certain pieces of music with which they became familiar while in the womb.

By the sixth month it seems that fetuses dream, as fibre-optic filming reveals rapid eye movements similar to those of dreaming adults. Some research implies that mother and baby exhibit simultaneous dreaming brain patterns. It is interesting to wonder what form and content fetal dreams may take. One possibility is that they, like adults, use dream time to digest and integrate waking experiences.

By the seventh month, internal organs are well developed. The baby has finger and toe nails, and the lungs are becoming capable of breathing air. Sexual differentiation of boys and girls, anatomically apparent since the twelfth week, is becoming complete.

Maternal Influences

The question whether the mother's thoughts and emotions can affect fetal wellbeing remains unanswered. Several studies indicate that maternal experience can be transmitted directly to the fetus. In one experiment by Benson, it was found that when women who rated themselves as anxious were played tapes of babies crying through headphones, fetal heart rate was affected, although obviously the baby could not hear the stimulus. Similarly, very early studies found changes in fetal heart rate following maternal distress. When monitored, maternal smoking was found to have a similar effect of increasing fetal heart rate – but so does a pregnant woman just *thinking* about having a cigarette. Salk's finding that babies in a nursery are soothed by a tape of regular maternal heartbeats, and become distressed at rates higher than eighty beats per second suggests that chronic maternal stress may affect the fetus, as may increased hormonal activity accompanying anxiety, distress, or over-exertion. The Fels longitudinal study found that in the course of their ten-year data collection, fetuses who were monitored before and after the occurrence of a severe emotional trauma to their mothers showed four to tenfold increase in activity, and about twenty-five beats per minute increase in heart rate. This persisted for several weeks, and well after the mother's manifestation of distress had disappeared. Compared to others, these fetuses were found to be hyperactive and irritable as babies, and some had severe feeding problems.

Paternal Influences

In different societies, beliefs vary as to the contribution of the parents in making a baby. In some it is assumed that mother merely incubates the 'homunculus', which is fully present in miniature in the father's seed. In others, the mother is seen to grow the body while the man contributes the soul. In yet others they each contribute to the formation of the child. A Jewish Talmudic view assumes the father's semen supplies the 'white substance' from which the bones, sinews, nails, brain, and whites of the eye are formed; the mother contributes the 'red substances' from which flesh, hair, skin and the iris are formed; God supplies the soul and breath, beauty of features, eyesight, hearing, speech, understanding, and discernment. A common fantasy, shared by expectant fathers in both developed and developing societies, is that of making contact with the unborn baby through intercourse – 'feeding' the baby with semen, thereby contributing to its growth.

Prenatal Loss

I never saw the features I had made,
The hands I had felt groping
For the life I had tried to give, and could not.
But still, I sometimes dream I hear it crying
Lost somewhere and unfed,
Shut in a cupboard, or lying in the snow,
And I search the night and call, as though to rescue
Part of myself from the grave of things undone.

Barbara Noel Scott, 'Stillbirth'

In our tendency to idealize maternity, it is not often acknowledged that about one in six confirmed pregnancies end in miscarriage, and possibly half of all conceptions. Around three quarters of all miscarriages occur in the first trimester, often coming as a shock to the woman who is blissfully unaware of the possibility of loss. Miscarriage disrupts a woman's fertile self-image, and is often accompanied by shame and a deep sense of ineffectiveness. If the baby has been conceived following infertility treatment, devastation is often accompanied by feelings of betrayal, hopelessness and anxieties about the artificial procedure as the source of the miscarriage. When death or destruction interrupt an established emotional trajectory of pregnancy, the trauma suffered by the psyche can feel as tangible as the physical one, also necessitating adapting to cessation of the momentum of pregnancy. However, due to social secrecy around loss and a taboo on mentioning death, it is not uncommon for a woman to feel unfairly singled out. This, as well as a sense of aloneness with the pregnancy in her body, isolates an expectant mother who has lost her baby. Being able to share her experience with other women who have suffered a miscarriage can mitigate some of the feelings of depression and failure (see Hey, Oakley).

The prevalent use of ultrasound as an initial screening technique for abnormalities and malformations seems to have the positive effects of personalizing the baby and possibly increasing prenatal bonding. Ironically, these same effects makes abortion or the threat of miscarriage more difficult to contemplate: 'There was this brilliant image of the baby on the screen', says a man whose pregnant partner is bleeding. 'It was still moving around as if to say "It's not so easy to get rid of me." The memory of seeing this little person alive on the TV screen just breaks my heart.'

The shock of threatened miscarriage is so dissonant with the optimism of pregnancy that early signs may be overlooked or ignored in the hope they will go away. In other cases, despite the absence of symptoms, a woman who is in touch with her own body may feel she is no longer pregnant, and investigation will reveal that the fetus has died, although expulsion may be delayed. Ultrasound confirmation of fetal life or death or a blighted ovum – when the baby does not develop – reduces uncertainty; however, emotional bewilderment continues as the shock waves register, before a process of grieving or rejoicing is instigated.

After a prolonged period of considerable bleeding, even a hopeful woman may reach an emotional watershed when she can no longer easily believe in the baby's viability. Her fierce desire to will the pregnancy to survive begins to alternate with gradual adjustment to the possibility, or even hope, of loss. In some cases the outcome is unclear, and the woman may alternate between twinges of hope with every movement of her gut, and a morbid fear of carrying a corpse or damaged baby within her. When pregnancy does continue, some women bounce back into optimism or denial, while others remain vigilantly concerned about the baby's survival and normality after this crisis, which may accompany the couple throughout the rest of the long wait for the birth, or even after.

A late miscarriage is particularly traumatic: the contractions sometimes simulate labour, and, if it occurs at home, the sight of a fully formed, recognizable baby is devastating. When expulsion is delayed, the sense of carrying around a dead body may be fraught with ambivalence, as the desire to retain the beloved baby conflicts with repulsion and fear. Late miscarriages which follow the experience of fetal movement, close bonding, and clear images of the baby are often accompanied by all the stages of mourning: shock, disbelief, anger, pangs of grief and searching for the baby, painful acceptance of the loss, and gradual recuperation, which may take many months to complete.

Despite having shared her pregnancy with a wider circle of acquaintances, miscarriage, like stillbirth, is often not regarded as a proper bereavement. The suffering woman and her partner are frequently denied opportunities to express grief by well-meaning friends and relatives, who reassure them with bland 'Never mind, you can have another', or shy away from the subject – or indeed from the couple.

Ectopic pregnancy concentrates many life events in one, each sufficient to create emotional turbulence: danger to the woman's life, post-operative pain and shock, miscarriage of the baby and possible loss of fertility, and hopes for another pregnancy. Having lost the baby, with all the attendant feelings of stunned grief, she may also feel guilt-ridden at not having provided a 'fruitful ground', angry ('he put his sperm in the wrong place'), and sorely cheated by not having had the emotional experience of knowing she was pregnant.

In a portion of cases, side by side with the live fetus an empty sac on the ultrasound screen indicates there had been twins, one of whom has aborted. In fact, we now know that in at least fifty per cent of twin pregnancies, one baby is lost, a technological phenomenon named 'the vanishing-twin syndrome'. This juxta-position of life and death, joy and mourning – like the painful paradox of life ending before it was begun – touch the family profoundly, and the live twin may continue unconsciously to be associated with the miscarriage.

In her inner experience, every miscarriage is a brush with death, not just close by, but inside the woman's own body. Nevertheless, as with other reproductive losses, a conspiracy of silence seems to descend after this major life event, which is often treated by others, and at times by the woman herself, as if nothing has occurred – a non-event. Despite the fact that miscar-riage touches off a whole host of emotions, grief, doubts, anxiety, or despair are sometimes regarded by medical staff and friends as excessive. The loss is not loss of 'the products of conception' – as euphemistically referred to in medical textbooks – or even loss of a baby alone; miscarriage causes disarray in the internal world as reality flings out all hopes and expectations invested in the baby, affecting the future as well as the present.

The need to understand what is felt to be a failure as well as a loss is magnified with recurrent miscarriages. Self-recriminations abound, as questions are raised in the woman's mind about her capacity to sustain a baby, and the goodness of her womb and placenta, triggering irrational ideas of being punished for past misdeeds, and guilt feelings about ambivalence in this pregnancy, or previous sexual encounters: in the absence of explanations, a self-condemning woman trying to make sense of her loss will clutch at old transgressions:

'I feel like a cork bobbing at the mercy of dark forces of inevitability', says Ruby, an older woman. 'There is no ar-bitrariness to fate. When I lost the baby, in my mind it was clearly a punishment for the abortion I'd had when I was nineteen. You can't get away from what you've done. It catches you up in the end.'

Others respond with anger, lashing out at anyone or thing that can be held responsible, including, at times, their partners. Magi-cal beliefs and superstitious avoidances are also common re-sponses to miscarriage, as they are to all inexplicable happenings. The woman whose pregnant process of introspection and fantasy was so rudely interrupted slowly begins a dazed recovery, usually in inverse ratio to her investment in the baby. However, precisely because of its nebulous nature and dearth of memories, mourning for the lost hopes and dreams that the baby represented is a long and complicated process, which may resurface in subsequent pregnancies or losses.

The terrible, unexpected loss of a child around birth is shocking in its curt finality. When a mother becomes aware that her baby has died before birth, she may feel a mixture of shock and despair, anguish and repugnance for the body turned corpse in her womb. Having to go through a painful, futile labour with no prize at its end is extremely distressing. When a woman begins labour with all the excitement of fulfilling the hopes of nine months waiting, stillbirth confronts her with a blank that cancels out all feeling. She and her birth partner may have been totally unprepared for the idea that anything could go wrong.

Many find their initial numbness grows into painful bewilderment, followed by rage that such a thing could happen. Seeking an explanation for the death, their anger is at times vented at the professionals who allowed it to occur, or seem not to care that it did. The staff, in turn, may have been so shocked by this uncommon happening that they whisk the baby away and leave the stunned parents to their own depleted resources.

In recent years, particularly following the work of psychoanalysts Stanford Bourne and Emannuel Lewis, an attempt has been made to replace the embarrassed silence about a 'non event' with constructive reactions. There has been a gradual change in attitude towards bereaved parents, and in many maternity units staff have been trained to provide compassionate care to help parents through the early stages of this equivocal time. Help hinges on an understanding that only a loss that is experienced can be mourned. Health care professionals are now coming to recognize that grief can be facilitated by reducing the fear of death. By gradually helping distressed parents to come closer to the dead baby, a midwife can enable parents to see, recognize, and possibly name their child if they wish. As the reality of the loss becomes tangible, memories are formed, and parents may wish to hold or dress the now more familiar baby, or ask for keepsakes, such as a lock of hair or name-bracelet. A photograph will be taken, so that parents who feel unable to spend time with the dead baby can do so when ready at a later stage.

When a late miscarriage, stillbirth or perinatal death occurs, parents often try to protect other children by hiding their grief. They overlook the fact that their young child is undergoing a mourning reaction of his or her own for the baby who was never brought home, and for the mother who was away. Lack of parental tears may be bewildering to the sad child, contributing to the precariousness of faith in the parent's trustworthiness as a source of security and safety.

Children need to talk about the terrible thing that has happened and why it could not be prevented; they need to make sense of death in their own terms and understand its ramifications. Bereaved siblings need to feel accepted, to have their fears allayed that death is unlikely to spirit them away, and that their own irrational but very real sense of blame is unfounded. Helping a child through his or her grief may provide the grieving mother and/or father with an outlet and solace for their own sense of loss.

Prenatal Testing – Abnormality

Threats of miscarriage and loss are quelled once viable gestation is safely underway. However, another reminder of uncertainty is embedded in antenatal care itself. Although the risk of abnormality is very low – around three per cent – almost all pregnant women undergo routine screening for congenital abnormalities and genetic disorders through a variety of more or less invasive techniques. While generally considered a beneficial advancement, and reducing anxiety in some expectant mothers, prenatal testing raises moral, ethical, and psychological issues.

For many women, contentment with pregnancy is disturbed from the early weeks by knowledge that prenatal screening brings with it an awesome dilemma. Faced with profound implications of the unknown, there is sometimes a temptation to comply blindly with expert advice. However, increasingly users of medical services are becoming more questioning, demanding to participate in making informed decisions on their own behalf. Pregnant women – defined as 'patients' although not ill; treated as incubators or bodies without feelings; yet conscious of having a responsibility towards the unborn child in addition to themselves – have been at the spearhead of this consumer movement. For some, prenatal tests enable them to follow the progress of the baby, and in the case of complications, such as possible prematurity or neonatal surgery, to prepare themselves for these. For others, they are an unbearable burden. Self-motivated decision-making is not without its price in anxiety:

'I've found myself thinking horrible thoughts, and unable to enjoy my pregnancy for a minute without feeling wretched and angry about having to make a decision whether to have the amniocentesis or not. The blood test was bad enough, but rather than reassure me it put the risk at eighty-two per cent because of my age. What if the amnio makes me miscarry this baby that I've waited for and suffered so much to conceive? And what if they say it is abnormal? I can't bear the thought of an abortion – but neither can I bear the thought of torturing myself with uncertainty for another five months', says Ruth.

'I'm tormented with the idea that if we had an abnormal baby I would be so ashamed I'd hide it away so as not to see the pitying, curious stares and awkwardness in people's faces. I want to love our baby, but it would be terrible being confronted with something I wanted to get rid of. At the same time I can't contemplate doing away with it', says Steve.

'All last week thinking about the tests I felt like hitting myself and the baby in my belly. I'm afraid I'd really hurt the baby or strangle it if it was born handicapped. I hated it for causing me so much trouble, and hated myself for feeling so selfish, and hated the doctors for giving me this terrible dilemma, and God for His moral values – and most of all I hated you for not giving me the answers and rescuing me from this incessant torment . . .', rages my young patient, giving voice to the feelings of many others in her situation.

For older women or those at risk, bonding may consciously be held in abeyance until test results are obtained. Amniocentesis, as a means of confirming suspicions raised by positive blood tests, can only be reliably conducted from the sixteenth to seventeenth weeks of pregnancy, with results often delayed for a further two weeks. Thus, for some women, decisions about possible termination have to be made as late as their fifth month of pregnancy. Furthermore, second trimester abortions become increasingly more difficult for both professionals and parents to contemplate, in parallel with survival of ever-younger premature babies:

'Everything has been dominated by the amniocentesis', says an older woman. 'It has been the biggest gamble of my life. I'm unable to deal with any other alternatives it presents except a healthy baby. I can't allow the baby to become real, and dreamed I was bathing a cooing, gurgling baby. Next thing I knew it had disappeared. I searched desperately, but it had been washed away down the drain as the plug came out, like a miscarriage or abortion.'

Fetal Malformation

One of the paradoxes of today is the emphasis on quality of life, which together with technological advances poses a possibility of selective termination of multiple or abnormal fetuses. Abortions because the baby has been discovered to be impaired or ill, are particularly poignant. By the time the diagnosis is made parental attachment has formed and parents may be aware of a terrible paradox: that abortion is recommended because prenatal corrective therapy is minimal, yet technological innovations are improving the chance of viability for increasingly younger, prematurely born and malformed babies.

The handling of the diagnosis and the period of decision-making often underplay the devastating bombshell effect of this situation. Scars, doubts, and, not uncommonly, depression follow termination. With the decision to abort, all the hopes, dreams, and fantasies surrounding the pregnancy are similarly aborted, and sometimes, parenthood itself:

'I knew something was wrong when the ultrasound technician stopped being chatty. Later she got the consultant and he explained to us about spina bifida, and that I would need to have an alpha-fetoprotein test to make sure. Those days of waiting were horrendous. I couldn't sleep, and would lie awake thinking I was carrying a monster, or going over every single thing I'd done in the early weeks that might have prevented the baby from growing properly. At first we were both so stunned we could hardly talk about it – then we couldn't talk about anything else. It was absolutely our worst nightmare come true. Once we agreed to terminate the pregnancy if the result was positive it became easier, although we still cried a lot and found it difficult to tell people, especially our parents, who'd been so thrilled that I was pregnant. By the time I had the abortion it was actually a relief. I honestly don't think I could go through all that again. It almost feels like a warning that we should have listened to our gut feelings and never tried to have a baby in the first place. But I still mourn the baby I will never have.'

Abortion of a wanted baby is accompanied by all the manifestations of mourning. In addition to accepting the loss of the baby, and psychologically reframing the future without the infant, the woman also experiences loss of pregnancy with all its attendant physical, social, and emotional processes and disillusionment with the natural process of gestation. The latter affects subsequent pregnancies. Even reassurance by the birth of a normal baby may not erase the deep scars left by this abortion. Some couples may avoid the necessary work of mourning by conceiving a replacement baby very soon, or refusing to contemplate another pregnancy.

For those who go on to have a handicapped baby, there are untold hardships and very little help. When parents have relied on technology, or have become beguiled by the promise of perfection in prenatal screening, the shock of producing an imperfect child may be punctuated with rage and disillusionment. For those who have knowingly chosen to go ahead or refused to have the tests, in addition to difficulties they may encounter unsympathetic reprehension.

With the availability of tests and social pressure to have terminations, coupled with potential breeding out of some disabilities, disapproval of handicap may be on the increase. Predictably, this will lead not only to greater prejudice and moralistic blame – 'Well, they could have aborted and didn't, so it's their own fault, isn't it?' – but to reduction in services for the incapacitated. The ethical issue remains one of who can decide and who determines the criteria, which life is and is not worth living.

Special Care Babies

Preterm births are defined as less than thirty-seven weeks gestation. Some preterm labours are spontaneous, others induced. About twenty per cent are multiple births, as about half of these are born prematurely. Other births are induced for reasons of maternal ill health or retarded growth in the baby.

Unexpected labour can be frightening when the woman is caught unawares, and the emotional trajectory of pregnancy is abruptly ended. Preterm birth seems to confirm her worst fears of being insufficiently good for the baby who, it is felt, is choosing to escape from inside her. Confusions arise as she is catapulted into the position of being a mother:

'I wasn't ready for my son. Intellectually I knew babies could be born as much as seven weeks early – it had happened to a friend of mine, but it never occurred to me that it could happen to me. I was given a due date and that was when my baby would be born. I'd even forgotten that I myself was born two weeks early . . . I suppose I didn't want to think of myself as born from my mother – she'd had two miscarriages following me and I felt somehow to blame for them, as if I'd left something behind inside her that killed them off. On one level, I must have expected I'd never be allowed to get away with having a baby myself. On another, I just took the doctor's word as gospel. So, when my waters broke at thirty-eight weeks, I didn't seem to realize what was happening. Nothing was ready, and I was emotionally unprepared for a birth or a baby.'

At first sight, the puny, almost transparent premature or ill baby is totally unlike the robust dream baby imagined during pregnancy. Often whisked away before the mother has a chance to become acquainted with her newborn, she feels alienated from the little scrap, heaving laborious breaths while wired-up to a life-sustaining incubator. Still reeling from the shock of unforeseen labour, the mother of a 'premie' is inevitably caught up in an emotional turmoil of interrupted pregnancy, guilt at having abandoned her baby to professionals and machinery, and an irrational sense of rejection and failure at having been unable to sustain the child who has chosen, or been forced, to leave her insufficiently nurturing womb.

The mother of an ill baby worries that she has contributed to her baby's condition, feeling guilty, too, about her ambivalence, shame and disappointment. The trauma continues as she finds herself physically separated, often by long draughty corridors, from the fruit of her pregnancy, and separated in feelings, unconsciously avoiding attachment in case the baby does not survive.

Anxious, exhausted, sore, and frumpish following her ordeal, she may feel intimidated and spare in the strange and often frightening atmosphere of the special care baby unit, where crisply uniformed nurses rush around competently pushing high-tech buttons, inserting tubes into fragile flesh and making life-saving decisions in response to bleeps and read-outs.

But her baby needs her. She is the human link between the biorhythms and pulsations that existed before this space-age nightmare. Her expressed milk can strengthen the baby, her soothing touch and reassuring voice familiar from pregnancy can help bind experiences too fragmenting and traumatic for the stressed infant to digest. And she needs the baby to complete the abruptly curtailed unfinished emotional business of her pregnancy. When the neonate is sufficiently recovered to be held outside the incubator, kangaroo-like, the mother (or the father, if her caesarean wound prevents it), may provide the warmth of skin-to-skin contact and familiar heartbeat by holding the baby inside their clothing, against the bare breast. Meanwhile warming their own hearts by allowing themselves to be touched by the child who has been held emotionally at bay.

Discussions with other parents of ill babies can help to promote self-help resources while alleviating the sense of desperate isolation and paranoid competition among those who feel death will arbitrarily take its share. Increased parental participation in baby-care, massage and stroking of the baby, phototherapy and tube-feeding on the mother's lap, dummies, diurnal light/dark patterns and simulated interuterine conditions, such as water beds, hammocks or sheep-skins within the incubators have all been linked to greater gains in low-birthweight babies. Once they leave the unit it often takes a long time for the family to re-establish the rhythms disrupted by the birth, and in some households these are never regained. In all these situations, family or individual therapy offers an opportunity to work through some of the traumatic events and emotional upheavals since the breaking of the waters, which may need to be talked through and processed verbally to become understood.

8
The Birth

'I wouldn't be so stupid as to pretend I have any idea of what Claudia was going through during the hours leading up to the birth. I goofishly hovered at the edges of her very own unique drama. It still didn't hit me that within hours we would have a baby: I vaguely felt I was immersed in some surreal soap-dream that constantly receded back into itself . . . She had an epidural. There was no shrieking agony or sweating exhaustion. Something was happening . . . a drifting, wafting hallucinatory journey towards a crazily peaceful and lovely, truthful climax that was far too cosmic and private and delicious and graceful a moment ever to write about . . . A moment that has become singly the most searing and beautiful and shimmering memory that I have. A great magnificent image . . . We had a baby; there she was and as far as I was concerned she was history. I was sopping and I didn't care less. I held her, trying to appear calm and composed on the outside, a shaking wreck inside . . .'

Paul Morley, 'On fatherhood'

Birth is an uncoupling. To some it is a welcome release from Siamese-like twinship, to others a wrench, a loss, an abandonment. There are as many variations as there are parturients in the world, but above them all, in each birth chamber, the archaic mother hovers, mumbling her curses or spreading her blessings. We are all born of woman, each of us exiled from and barred re-entry to that home which in the anxiety of severence and separation has become the seat of uncanny reverberations.

Observers and birth carers alike behold with awe and dread the birthing body of the mother, and, depending on their personal capacity to tolerate the pull towards the heart of darkness, will trust the process of two labouring as one towards their ultimate division, try to control it, or else defensively escape from the scene. Others address this anxiety by attempting to tame the primeval process through active intervention.

Choices – Venue and Attendants

For each woman and her baby the birth is a momentous, once-off life event. Although safety is a priority, she is also keen for the birth to be as personally meaningful as possible. Reliving the experience of the birth and infancy of a baby at various later points in their lives, many mothers have felt that a crucial opportunity of reconciliation with an alienated part of themselves was missed. The sheer enormity and primitive quality of the birth experience grants it a power that can have either reparative or harmful ramifications. Endorsing a woman's trust in her own capacities, and increasing the opportunities for taking meaningful decisions based on real information can mean the difference between a thwarted or passive experience, and one of exuberant empowerment.

In Western societies, where there is greater variety of practices, a woman's personal choices of birth venue and attendants are crucial in ensuring a good fit between her expectations and the actual experience. While psycho-social circumstances and physical conditions may dictate her decision, unconscious factors may determine her wishes and fears.

Like birth practices, the place of birth reveals a great deal about a society's values. In many societies birth takes place in seclusion, or in a special place designed for it. In others, birth may be regarded as a social event accessible to many and celebrated by the community. In a few, such as Holland, it is an intimate, wholesome event within the mother's own bedroom. The place of birth is determined by fantasies surrounding the birth, whether regarded as a dangerous, potentially contaminating event, a semi-sacred or numinous happening, an auspicious occasion, or a physical crisis. In our own society, changing attitudes over the last century have altered the intimate emotional event of yore into a public, medical event, centralized among strangers. Removing the parturient out of the security of her home and community, she is transplanted to an institution of morbidity and high technology.

But it need not be so. One of the most untrammelled births I have seen was not a homebirth but located in a small homely birth centre, attached to a hospital in a medium-sized town in southern Sweden. Filmed by a fixed video camera, labour took its course in the same warm, subdued, spacious room, with snack-making facilities and low double bed, where all the woman's antenatal checkups had taken place. The midwife sat unobtrusively in a corner of the room until called, leaving the male partner, dressed only in underpants, to support, hold, caress and massage his naked wife as she swayed and rocked, pendulous breasts and rotund belly smoothly changing positions as she surrendered herself to an internal gyroscope, gliding from kneeling to leaning, all-fours to squatting, reclining through sitting to standing, throughout the long night – *pas de deux* in slow motion, heads together, swaying and moaning, grasping and sweating in unison until, almost without warning, as the woman advanced to second stage where he could not follow her – the 'two-backed beast' finally split apart. With uncanny plaining howls such as I have heard only from unself-conscious birthing or bereaved women who have lost all sense of worldly awareness while relinquishing their loved one, the woman bore down. Gripping her kneeling man's upper arms with ruthless strength as she squatted and pushed against gravity, with a final keening cry her bursting perineum gave up its treasure, a fitting orgasmic end to the ten-moon-long process of slow ripening since that original lovemaking that began it all.

The main criteria in the choice of a birth place is whether a woman feels accepted and secure, and trusts her baby will be safely delivered and cared for. It is preferable to consider labour options during pregnancy, at a time when the mother can think in a relaxed manner about her priorities, and formulate a birth plan that reflects her personal choices within the limits of safety.

In this affirmed state, self-confidence reduces both the shock and sense of failure experienced by many women who are caught short by the unexpected less-than-perfect eventualities, such as emergency Caesareans, or a premature baby in need of special care.

Unconscious Factors

The paradox of pregnancy is never so apparent as in the fundamental birth dilemma: when the woman – supremely powerful in her goddess-like capacity to bring a new life into being – is also threatened by the crucial human responsibility of bringing that life safely to fruition. At this threatening time we tend to revert and there may be an internal gravitation towards a soothing mother figure, or to an image of paternalistic benevolence, which promises to protect both her and the baby, calling the Oedipal child in her into strong, medicalized arms. Even women who have spent their lives fighting for control over their bodies and their right to autonomy may feel incapacitated by the fear of loss of that control. To some of these, active birth is the answer; to others, the idea of streamlined, technological birth offers hope of retaining a shred of dignity in the face of emotional disarray.

With a home birth, good practice means the pregnant woman has time to get to know and build a trusting relationship with carers, and is given sufficient information to make choices and freedom to ask for more information when anxious. However, although she is mistress of the place of birth, and the midwife a guest, a home birth does not mean the woman will automatically feel relaxed and prepared for labour. She too must confront her fear of pain, and anxieties about bodily incompetence and emotional reluctance to go through with it. She needs space to contemplate her own internal resources and stamina in order to marshall these towards the labour.

> 'I can't bear the thought of a hospital birth – that clinical atmosphere, and everyone bossing me about. I want to be comfortable in my own home, taking my time to find out what my body can do, without interference. If something goes wrong, the hospital is only a short ride away.'

A home birth may be as natural as breathing for some women, but seem foolhardy for others. A woman may wish to give birth in a high-tech setting that can take care of all eventualities: her internal doubts advocate placing herself in the hands of professionals, who will tell her exactly what to do, thereby relieving her of responsibility and possible blame.

> 'Birth belongs to the doctors and midwives. The thought of a home birth to me is ghastly – all by myself at home with a midwife and no medical equipment! I wouldn't trust myself. I don't feel anyone has much control over what happens in labour, and I'm frightened that if I lose control so will my partner, and he won't be strong enough to help me through.'

A smaller, more intimate setting may be the choice of another woman, echoing an internal sense of there not being enough care to go round. Others prefer a domino arrangement, or early discharge, or home birth with an independent midwife. However, many women fail to explore their options for fear of being criticized for wanting something special.

Birth is the culmination of a woman's long ordeal of pregnancy: she is entitled to express her wishes and anxieties without it being regarded as neurotic weakness or petulance. It is she who will experience the labour along with her baby, and she who will have to live with the consequences for years to come.

Wise Women and Carers

By contrast to our own, in traditional communities pregnant women are wrapped in a time-embroidered shawl of familiar customs, each woman experiencing pregnancy as did her mother, and often her grandmother before her. Through the years, she has been ripened for the birth of her own child with each successive birth in her extended family group, and since childhood has heard about many labours in juicy detail, and possibly observed some. Bearing a sibling or cousin on her own hip since she was a young girl, she was often handed responsibility for mothering smaller babies and is equally familiar with neonates.

By contrast, the breakup of the extended family in Western industrialized societies has resulted in our isolation in nuclear households. These often preclude intimate contact between blood relatives, with consequent loss of female lore and family traditions of pregnancy and childbirth by the jettisoned new mother:

'In my family in the North [of England], I spent my childhood overhearing the women recounting their bodily experiences, from menstrual difficulties to blow-by-blow, gory accounts of births. All my aunties take it for granted that they are surrogate mums and built-in-babyminders for all the cousins, supplying the crib and cuddles as well as material assistance, physical support, and free advice. By coming to London, I've removed myself, and although I've tried to reconnect with my origins, that kind of close warmth is localized to village life – it can't stretch down the motorways', says Jane, a barrister, having her first baby in her mid-thirties.

'No one talks about their fears. The books only say that fear increases anxiety, but don't acknowledge that there's a good

reason to fear', says Daniel's mother, in her thirty-eighth
week of pregnancy. 'It *is* frightening to live with uncertainty.
It's all so very real, and I'm alone and scared. I'm scared of
going into labour when I'm on my own with Daniel. There
really is a case for a family all living under one roof. I'm so
ungainly, and Daniel's so heavy. And I keep forgetting or
dropping things. If I was surrounded by caring people, my
pregnant absentmindedness would seem endearing, but on my
own, with all the responsibility for the household on my
shoulders, I find it frightening . . .'

Good care caters to the whole woman and the whole process.
One of the difficulties now recognized and beginning to be addressed is the *fragmentation* of care, with a variety of specialist
professionals each providing aspects of ante- and postnatal
healthcare. This differs from the traditional approach of continuity of care – the wise woman who acts as a guide and intermediary between past and future, new mother and society,
natural and supernatural – protecting both women and fetus
during pregnancy and acting as a bridge to her new status.
   The traditional birth attendant is likely to be an older, respected member of the community, experienced in childbearing
and caring, who, in addition to midwifery skills, usually presides
over matters of fertility, contraception, conception, abortion,
gestation, nutrition, birth, lactation and spiritual purification. In
our system, the combination of a multitude of specialists in the
context of a male-dominated institution fragments the trans-
ferences. This convolutes and dilutes strong feelings and deters
them from being invested in a single maternal figure, who could
help a woman cross the watershed between herself as her
mother's child, to becoming her child's mother.

In recent years, mothers and midwives alike have become involved in a campaign to reinstate female care, individual choice,
and safe homebirths, and particularly to acknowledge the pri-
macy of emotional needs. While monitoring physiological processes, few Western health carers encourage clients to express
their feelings. Indeed, midwives sometimes admonish the labouring woman for making too much noise. The quintessential
female process of gestation offers a special chance for caregivers
to re-establish maternal values of relatedness and nurturing

between and among women, with emphasis on continuity and integrity of the whole trajectory from preconception to child-care. Most antenatal clinics neglect a golden opportunity to facil-itate communication among pregnant women in their care, either in organized discussion groups or informal interchange. Child-birth education classes tend to provide varieties of exercises and breathing and relaxation techniques, but rarely explore the psy-chological dimensions of bodily anxieties and emotional con-cerns, which, if unvoiced, can contribute to labour obstructions. Given an opportunity to express their feelings – in group meet-ings with other pregnant women or in psychotherapy – expectant mothers feel tremendous relief at finding their uncer-tainties shared by others with similar doubts and fears.

Medical Institutions

I am writing this in a small airport in China, awaiting a plane back to London. The birth I filmed yesterday brought home to me forcibly that whatever our cultural differences – and there are a great many between us and the Chinese – the event of birth is a common denominator: the labouring woman, her contracting womb, dilating cervix, hardening belly, rounding perineum, crowning head, and sudden gush of amniotic liquid; then that translinguistic command – 'Wait!' – and then – 'Push!' – followed by the slow emergence of the head, and then the slithering rush of a twisting, slippery body.

These are the same the world over, yet even among the similarities, differences set in. Society puts its print on the newborn before he or she ever reaches the mother's breast. In the case of the baby girl I saw born yesterday in a Chinese university teaching hospital, after the cut cord was clamped, one of the presiding midwives carried her by arm and leg to the suction-table and slapped her feet as her first cry was followed by no breath. Finally, bundled and labelled, she was shown to her exhausted mother. The silent parturient – head lolling back downwards towards the floor, as she lay feet-first on the sloping, narrow birth table – opened her resigned eyes and looked at the carefully wrapped female parcel. Alone des-pite the four attending midwives, flat on her back, legs apart and inserted in burlap sausages against the bitter cold in the unheated room, she patiently awaited the afterbirth and stitching and her family's disappointment. The baby was whisked away to a nursery, where thirty other identically wrapped babies lay in cots. In China, 1.7 million girl babies are aborted, abandoned or vanish each year.

In previous generations, many people were conceived, born, and eventually died in the same bed, in the same household, surrounded by family and the familiar objects of a lifetime. Today, birth and death often take place in institutions, in the presence of strangers. Most women have had little previous contact with hospitals, or only occasional visits associated with morbidity and casualty. Mothers intending to give birth in hospital worry about the reception they and the baby will receive. Compounding the horror of being in pain in strange surroundings, a woman fears disorientation. Worried she may lose her bearings away from the comforting smell and familiar confines of home, she dreads abrogating her body's management to people she does not know or trust. She has qualms about being intimidated by the clinical atmosphere of the delivery room, wondering whether she might lose her self-confidence under conditions of extreme pain; start screaming and never stop; or not feel free to experience her own feelings under the dual taskmasters of internal pressures of having to be 'good' and 'act sensibly', and external commands from well-meaning, uniformed strangers: 'Last time it was like being on a potty and being told to "Push!" I cringe when I think of the humiliation of not being able to perform according to their expectations.'

She dreads finding herself on an escalating roller-coaster of interventions which lead to each other and cascade beyond control, allowing her no, space to catch her breath or recapture a sense of herself and what she has wished for. Her conflict may lie in wanting to use the resources available to minimize any risks to herself and her baby, yet afraid of being sucked into a technological birth that allows little freedom for personal desires:

'I don't want any interventions, but I'm afraid they'll insist. Last time, as soon as they ruptured my membranes the contractions became so strong so suddenly, I had to have an epidural, and then I couldn't feel the urge to push. I ended up having a huge episiotomy and forceps delivery and poor Sarah was born looking like a monster – her head had large lumps and bruising. It took me weeks to fall in love with her.'

Indeed, some hospitals do demand conformity, introducing routine practices intended to increase 'efficiency', sometimes equated with rapid delivery. Offended by such policies, pregnant women have demanded changes which make concessions to individual needs. Personalized birth plans and staff protocols have been instituted, and routine procedures have been queried including shaving, strirrups, membrane-rupture, drips, lithotomy, episiotomies, and fetal-scalp monitoring and suction. However, changing the underlying assumptions and a deeply ingrained ethos has been a slow process as it is in the nature of institutions to defend professionals against empathic involvement. In the case of birth, these emotions are intensely personal, and aggravated by chronic tension and exposure to pain and intimacy. Elliott Jaques has shown how institutions tend to develop mechanisms to defend their familiar practices, and to protect personnel from being flooded by unmanageable anxieties, which, by distribution of responsibility and standardization of practice, reduces personal initiative and involvement to the minimum.

Different Orientations

Women differ in their needs. Generally speaking, whereas women of the Facilitator orientation will desire a natural birth, often at home, Regulators will want a civilized one, and Reciprocators tend to go for an active birth. These differences are not whims, but reflect deep unconscious beliefs about the birth process.

To the Facilitator, labour is an exciting, powerful process to which she and the baby must surrender in order to be reunited. Her main fear is interference: induction before the baby is ready; escalation, disrupting the spontaneous, synchronized rhythmicity, and intrusion into the orgasmic intimacy of their division and greeting. Given a choice, the Facilitator desires a home birth. If this is not possible, all she wants is a midwife who will watch over her until she is ready to draw her baby out herself and suckle him or her before the cord is even severed. She avoids any separation from her baby, and may choose an early discharge if in hospital.

To the Regulator, labour is a medical event; an inescapable, painful crisis inflicted upon her, to be endured with minimal discomfort by using all the means at her disposal to shorten and anaesthetize the procedure. Choosing a hospital birth, she tends

to admit herself early in labour, which may lead to various intervention procedures, such as artificial rupturing of the membranes. Lacking faith in her body's primordial knowledge of
childbirth, her main concern is to retain maximum control. A
fetal monitor offers her information about the progress of labour
and offsets her anxieties. Most of all, a Regulator fears being
embarrassed and exposed during labour. Unlike the Facilitator,
the Regulator welcomes giving birth among strangers, and the
knowledge that she will never need see them again. Far from
immediate bonding, she wants to make the baby's acquaintance
gradually, having been given time and space to recuperate from
the ordeal of the birth; if the hospital has a nursery, for example,
she might wish to have the baby sleep there on the first night.

The Reciprocator treats the birth as a natural process whereby
the baby is ready to take its place in the world outside. She might
oppose the use of pain-killing drugs, but may make use of gas
and air, or a self-controlled battery-operated transcutaneous
nerve stimulation system (TENS), which blocks pain signals.
Aware of the unpredictable nature of labour – with possible
unforseen complications which may necessitate intervention –
even with a home birth she prefers to be within reach of emergency equipment. She finds the actual birth of the baby exhilarating and is keen to get to know her baby.

Questions Without Answers

We have all been subject to that journey from the inner space of a
female body; slithering through a ripened cervix, expelled head-
first or extracted, and lifted out into the light, before being cut
adrift from the supporting lifeline as we gasp for air. Awaiting
her day, the swollen-bellied woman of each generation is confronted afresh by the awesome challenge of birth and severance,
this time from the inside out. As the delivery date approaches,
birth anxieties proliferate and primal preoccupations are basic.

There is only one certainty about birth: what is in must come
out. Throughout the long months of her pregnancy, questions
gather as the baby gets larger, occupying her waking hours, fantasies, and dreams; what is 'it' that is developing inside her? Who
will emerge? How will she feel once she is emptied?

If she has not experienced birth before, the idea of uterine
contractions propelling the baby down the birth canal, and the

massive dilation of her vagina to enable the large-headed baby to come out of her little hole are unimaginable and fill her with dread. Cloacal fantasies are revitalized, as are wishes and dreams that birth could take place through a magical opening: the navel, or by proxy through osmosis.

To escape her disturbing fantasies, she turns to the experts. They try to describe it, telling her it is like expelling a large grapefruit or melon – but why should that make it more believable, not having had the experience of excreting whole fruit? Others say it is the most exhilarating experience ever – but how can that be so if it hurts? Birth educators tell her that if she breathes correctly and does what she has been taught, everything will be all right – but how can she be sure to remember everything when the time comes?

Rightly, she concludes that birth is an extraordinary happening, and that the uniqueness of each mother's experience makes generalizations impossible. Throughout all the long months of waiting, uncertainty prevails and she remains mystified: what will happen? When will it happen? How will she know it is happening? Will she be with someone, or alone? Where will she be – at home, on the bus, in the street?

Sometimes it feels as if the baby will keep on getting bigger until her body stretches to its limits and bursts at the seams. Other times, she has a horror that the baby might come before its time, before her time, before time, after time – never. So many unanswered questions; so many answered and still unknown.

In the absence of experienced older women, many expectant mothers, worrying they will not know when labour has begun, may take flight to hospital at the first indication of contractions. If she has mistaken strong Braxton-Hicks pangs for labour, however, she might be told on arrival that she is in false labour and sent home, often without the explanation that these irregular practice contractions are preparatory labour, giving her warning and time to rest up. Another woman may ignore her period-like cramps, and even when in established labour may find it difficult to assess the point at which she should go to hospital. Labour that begins with a show can be frightening, coloured by an irrational belief that once the mucous 'plug' is removed the baby might fall out. The waters breaking may increase self-doubts, as a childish shame at wetting her pants is revived – at the very moment when she is about to be initiated into the 'grown up' womanly world. Even a woman who has had a positive experience of labour before will experience some trepidation, resenting her powerlessness in determining the time and place of onset of labour, and worrying she might misidentify the signs.

In the transition from daughterhood to motherhood, a pregnant woman often unconsciously looks to her birth attendants to offer her emotional support, and to provide the maternal reassurance that she is permitted to enter the realm of the mothers, and allowed to have and keep her baby. Unless she feels free to settle into the rhythmic process of her own labour in her own right, she may be unconsciously compelled to re-enact her mother's or a significant other's labour – as told or imagined – or else she may abrogate body ownership to the experts' management.

Throughout the hours of labour, as contractions increase in duration, intensity, and frequency, the woman's emotions also peak and ebb – rising to momentary panic or rage at the height of a contraction, followed by release and sometimes blissful intervals of floating calm between. In the course of labour her feelings may range from elation and abandonment to anxiety, irritation, weepiness and despair, particularly towards or during transition.

Despite being centered deep inside herself, the woman in labour often has a heightened awareness of non-verbal messages, picking up vibrations of tenderness, acceptance, or disapproval in those around her. This sensitivity, however, is not necessarily reciprocated, and she is often treated matter-of-factly by professionals who measure the 'efficiency' of her progress, or those who, unable to bear with her – or to bear their own feelings of helplessness – feel impelled to 'do something' to augment labour, such as rupturing the membranes 'to get things going', or, unable to sit it out with her, leave her to her own resources.

Conversely, although there is a wish by the woman to be telepathically understood and physically cherished at this time, even a caring attendant will probably need some verbal instruction when she or he fails to anticipate her needs.

Journey to the Exterior

'It's all over, the baby has been born and my ordeal is at last at an end. I have risen from my bed and am gradually entering life again, but with a constant feeling of fear and dread about my baby and especially my husband. Something within me seems to have collapsed and I sense that whatever it is will always be there to torment me . . . for I am frightened by the womb's vulgar love for its offspring. . . .'

The diaries of Sofia Tolstaya,
wife of Leo Tolstoy, 14 July 1863

Birth hails a new journey for baby and parents: from psychic into external reality. With the final push of expulsion, the baby's first cry calls the new mother out of her intensely focused inner preoccupation. Opening her eyes, she is faced with a moulded, bluish, scrawny creature – quite unlike the pink, chubby-faced cherub of her dreams. Tentatively greeting the little stranger, new mother and father must relinquish an imaginary baby to make way for this real one, whose looks, feel, and sometimes gender, are not what was anticipated at all.

The phasing out of home births has meant that few adults in Western societies have ever seen newborn babies at close range. They may appear disappointing, and different from the smooth, two-week-old newborns in the movies. In real life, babies tend to be less well covered with flesh, and the head might have become moulded by the birth process, distorting its shape. Hair, if there is any, is matted, wet, usually blood-streaked, and darker than it will ultimately be. Following a forceps delivery, swellings on the head and bruise marks on the cheeks look alarming to parents, although they subside within a few days. The baby's features may be somewhat squashed, and ruptured blood vessels, due to the pressure of birth, cause skin discolourations and red streaks in the eyes. Rashes and reddened eyelids are common, as are other fading birthmarks such as red patches above the nose bridge and on the back of the neck colloquially called 'stork bites' said to be caused by the bill of the stork who brings the baby. Immediately after the birth, the newborn is covered in white vernix and blood from the labour. She or he may have some fine bodily hair. The sight of the genitals often cause consternation, as in both sexes they are swollen, and look disproportionate to the little scrawny body. Breast enlargement and hardening is common in both boys and girls due to maternal hormones, and some babies produce fluid known as 'witches milk'.

Although rarely practised for practical reasons, a day or two after the baby is born it is of great benefit to the mother to re-meet one of the people present at the birth, for a kind of debriefing chat that will enable her to ask questions and fill the gaps in her memory, or reduce confusion by confirming details she cannot believe actually occurred:

'It was only when we got to meet the paediatrician at the three-month checkup that I realized my baby's condition was not due to something I did to her during the birth, but that she was in distress because the cord had been round her neck. I'd spent all this time in such a state of guilty anguish – I could hardly hold her for fear of damaging her', says the mother of a baby who had spent some days in an intensive care unit.

Episiotomy

It is a rare woman who does not cringe at the thought of an episiotomy – being cut in that most private and tender area of her anatomy. In addition to physical fears, the psychological connotations of this threat loom large as, awaiting birth, the pregnant woman rages helplessly at the possible infliction of an episiotomy, dreading the humiliation, outrage, and pain of being cut against her will, seemingly punished for thinking she can get away with wanting a baby without being scarred for life by the experience of having had one.

Psychoanalysts speak of infantile castration anxieties. Like female circumcision, episiotomy is a reality. Compared to anxieties about painful hours of labour and birth, this concern is a long-term one. Her genital area will never return to its previous state. Self-esteem and body image are violated by an inflicted procedure which proclaims disbelief in her ability to complete the birthing without artificial intervention. A woman is concerned about damages to her body and its psychological effects on her feminine sexuality and selfhood. In addition to trepidation about birth-battering of her internal organs and body orifice – which may be so great as to cause some women to want a Caesarean – there are often anxieties as to whether, once sewn up, her vaginal opening and perineum will ever feel the same again, and how the scarring will affect her love-life:

'I'm so afraid that under the effect of pain in childbirth, I'll get very aggressive and be seen not to be handling it well', says one pregnant Regulator. 'What I really want is a Caesarean. I'd rather a small incision in my stomach which is robust and hardy than have my insides ripped apart and be manhandled and cut in my most delicate parts.'

For readers about to give birth, I can offer no reassurance. Although newly trained midwives are re-learning old delivery techniques, episiotomy is said to be still fairly prevalent in many hospitals. However, it can be avoided through the parturient's sheer obstinate determination to remain intact. The cut itself and suturing is usually relatively painless, as it is preceded by a local anaesthetic and the stretched perineum is naturally numbed. However, the sound and feel of scissors are unpleasant at the climactic moment of birth.

Once the anaesthetic wears off, the perineum is bruised and sore. Simple functions may become terrifyingly strange as the stitches make sitting down painful for a week or more, peeing burns, and having a bowel movement can be accompanied by intense pain, and (usually unfounded) fear that straining will cause the stitches to tear the skin.

Many mothers find the healing process can be speeded up by warm salt-baths and hair-dryer. However, the wrenching pain and basic discomfort at the very time when physical demands on her body are at their peak is maddeningly inappropriate.

'It's insane. As daft as a trainer cutting an athlete's achilles tendon to make the ankle more flexible, and then sending him on a marathon', says an irate mother.

Although a lot of women find little difference in the elasticity of the vagina once the episiotomy has had a chance to heal properly, others feel persistent tenderness or hypersensitivity along the scar for months or years. Complaints of decreased lubrication, stress incontinence, or pain on intercourse are common, and a few experience permanent loss of sphincter flexibility. However, even in the absence of physical symptoms, unconscious fantasies accompany the woman's rage at having been impaired and her sense of violation:

'Nobody ever mentioned stitches or the bleeding. That consultant wrecked me. I felt damaged and unclean, mutilated by his brutality like a bloody rape victim, and have not felt the same about myself since', says a mother some years later.

Not all women are as articulate in their expression of outrage, and some accept the episiotomy side-effects as part of the inevitable reduction of sexuality due to maternity. Some partners, however, may experience horror at this 'barbaric' act ('they sliced her open') constituting an, often unjustifiable, intrusion into their sexual intimacy. Ironically, obstetricians often justify the episiotomy on the phallocentric grounds of tightening a slack vagina. Although often not disclosed to the birth attendants, for women who have actually been abused in childhood or raped, any genital violence, including internal examinations, episiotomy and forceps delivery is traumatic. Indeed, some women first recall repressed sexual abuse under the impact of the birth experience, or in its aftermath.

Caesarean Section

Over the past twenty years, the rate of Caesarean section in the UK has risen dramatically, from less than five per cent of all deliveries to about fifteen per cent. In the United States, Caesarean section is now the most frequently performed major operation, totalling nearly thirty per cent of births. Reasons for the change appear to be related to: fear of litigation; prior Ceasarean section (both particularly in the United States); breech and pre-term births being seen as automatic indications; and varying criteria for prolonged labour or fetal distress. In England the majority of women have a vaginal delivery following a C-section.

From the woman's point of view, a distinction must be made between the emotional impact of an emergency Caesarean, and a planned operation. Even in the case of 'elective' Caesarean, however, the news that her pregnancy must end artificially may come like a bolt from the blue. Hearing the doctor's verdict, a woman and her partner may feel as if harsh reality has overtaken them. The implications of the news may take time to sink in, as fond dreams of a perfect birth fall by the wayside. They may feel cheated and appalled, being singled out when all their expectant acquaintances are looking forward to an 'ordinary' birth.

To some Regulator mothers, a Caesarean may seem like the perfect answer: knowing the date of the birth in advance, planning one's life accordingly, and having the baby 'removed' – rather than having to go through all that unpredictable and painful stuff ('You roll in, have an injection, and wake up to find your baby beside you – it seems ideal!'). Bypassing vaginal delivery may feel like a relief for rape or abuse survivors, for whom the genital zone is hypersensitized.

Some women may feel that working towards a set date is more frightening because of the fears and uncertainties about the surgery and its outcome. Others who fear damaging the baby during birth may be relieved to have responsibility taken from them, and to be given the newborn unmoulded by the birth process. On a practical level, like all crises, recovery is aided by briefing and information. If the baby is to be born prematurely some of the concerns about its wellbeing may be discussed with the paediatrician before the birth, and a visit to the neonatal special care unit can familiarize parents-to-be with a place which often seems frightening in the vulnerable period immediately after the birth. The hiatus thus can be utilized to alleviate anxieties rather than exacerbate them. Like all surgical operations, the more factual information she has about the procedure and the more time to absorb this and ask for explanations, the less the mother's fantasies will run riot, and the better prepared she will feel.

Unexpected premature labour in itself is shocking, filling the woman with questions about why her baby wants to leave her before term. An emergency Caesarean may feel like an additional betrayal, mother and/or baby being cheated out of a natural birth. If following prolonged labour a Ceasarean is found to be necessary, the exhausted woman may find the ordeal particularly frightening. The woman might wish to ask for the midwife who has attended her labour to accompany her to the theatre and remain with her throughout, thus providing continuity and reassurance. Others may feel relief:

'There was this terrible period when I couldn't get her out. It was so frightening. I felt she was stuck because she was too scared. I was afraid to push, and didn't want them to pull her out with forceps because I dreaded her getting squashed or me being hurt inside. When they eventually decided to do a Caesarean, I remember a sense of great relief, as if the die had been cast, everything was soon to be revealed, and the anguish of waiting and trying was almost over.'

Even a well-prepared woman may experience unexpected psychological reactions, which are exacerbated if she is unprepared for the long-term consequences of a Caesarean section. The early weeks with her baby may be problematic as she has to recuperate from a major operation while tending to someone else's basic needs. Cautioned to be careful in lifting and carrying, the mother is restricted in her care of the baby, and may find walking or even laughing painful for some time.

Days or even months following the euphoria and gratitude of an at-risk baby having been born safely, a deep sense of loss or failure may suddenly crop up, accompanied by a feeling of having had a baby without giving birth. Not having watched the baby emerge from within her, a common reaction following Caesarean section under a general anaesthetic is the fear of having been given the wrong baby. Cheated of the birth she had planned, the quick transition from pregnancy to the baby leaves her feeling robbed of saying goodbye to her fantasy baby. Her body image may be so altered by the birth and/or postoperative pain that she feels unable to reconcile her old body with the new, scarred one, which will forever remind her of this birth.

A woman may blame herself for not giving birth normally, or feel angry and physically violated by the surgeons who intervened and never gave her a chance. She may resent her partner for allowing it to happen, or blame herself for not resisting psychological pressure and insisting on having the vaginal birth she had wanted: 'They said that terrible phrase, "It's best for the baby." I accepted their verdict, but often wonder whether I should have tried harder before giving in and giving up.' She may feel she has let her baby down, depriving him or her of a birthright to struggle towards life, and herself of the experience of pushing her internal baby out into the world. Unresolved, such regrets may persist for years.

It is important that the mother realize these feelings are not unique to women who have had Caesareans. When mothers look back at the birth, most feel there are aspects of labour they wish had been different, or that they had not done the best by their babies during the birth or its aftermath. Poignant regrets are part and parcel of the difficult emotional task of every thoughtful mother who finds that reality can never be as perfect as she would like it to be for her infant. For some women, the Caesarean experience is made more satisfactory by having an epidural, so she is present at the birth and able to hold and feed her baby immediately after. Another woman may feel squeamish about the idea of being cut open while fully awake, even if she feels no pain, and prefers to have her partner receive the baby and look after him or her until she comes to from the anaesthetic. Such fathers, who have had the experience of being custodian of the birth and the first to hold the newborn baby, tend to feel unusually attached to and protective of that baby.

The process of parental adaptation may take days or weeks, as the baby's features emerge and become familiar. Many new parents feel cheated of their dream, disappointed with this baby they have been given on a non-returnable basis. Initial responses may be defensively numbed. In their study of 120 women giving birth, Kay Robson and Channi Kumar found that close to fifty per cent of new mothers reported indifference as the main predominant emotional reaction on holding their newborns.

Nevertheless, as Marshall Klaus has demonstrated, bonding may be accelerated in the first hour or two after the birth, as a cascade of interactive processes begin to unfold. In many cases, babies of mothers who have taken no analgesic drugs during labour are more alert during the first ninety minutes than they will be for some days. For many mothers, this is a time of heightened receptivity before the euphoria of birth has worn off – although others may be too exhausted to care about anything except recuperating. Even on the delivery table, the crawling reflex of a baby lying on the mother's tummy, or the little stepping movements when he or she is held in a standing position may delight parents with a glimpse into the future.

Birth is the end of one journey and the beginning of another. Although early deprivation and emotional trauma undoubtedly become the source of ongoing vulnerabilities in adults, psychic development and healing continues throughout life, as do interpersonal influences and stressors. We do not step-wise outgrow our past in discrete developmental stages, but lifelong emotional processes continue, building upon accrued intersecting 'layers', reworking with previous issues, and revising earlier schematic versions. A wide range of dynamic experiences, interlaced with psychic configurations of self and other coexist within our internal worlds, changing kaleidoscopically as different aspects come together or break away. For those who can grasp them, pregnancy and early parenthood offer rich emotional opportunities for redressing old imbalances. History is recycled for the mother by juxtaposition of the baby in the womb with the baby in her mother's womb, and projection of her wishes, hopes, fears and fantasies into a dream-child receptacle. The first postnatal weeks are not merely a period of learning to cope with a new baby, but a passionate confrontation with a being that has been inside her and knows her body from within, whose smell and feel is deeply evocative and stirs up archaic residues from infancy in both her and the father. Gradually these primary identifications are relinquished to be replaced by recognition, compassion, and acceptance – which are the birthright of each family member.

9
Different Approaches to Parenting – Facilitators Regulators and Reciprocators

'I thought I'd get straight back to my original identity immediately,' complains Lisa, three months after having her baby, 'but my body shows I'm a mother. I'm damned tired all the time, and my work capacity is up the creek.'

'There's a conspiracy to believe you can get back to normal,' says Maggie, holding her plump seven-week-old daughter, 'but you're no longer the same person. The reality is that life is different with a baby. It's irrevocable.'

'My mother treats me as if there's been *no* change. She just doesn't see me as a responsible adult. She can't bear having no control over how I'm bringing up her grandchild', Vicky says sadly, stroking her sleeping son's hair.

'I know what you mean', says Colleen. 'Now she's coming here, I have this overriding desire to get rid of my mother. I've always felt she didn't mother me as much as I'd like, but now, when I'm anxious and insecure with the baby, I'm filled with dread at her visits. She thinks she's coming to be helpful, but she really can't believe I can cope.'

'My image of my mother has changed', muses Maggie. 'I dedicated my life to not being martyred like her. But I'm much more like her than I thought . . .'

'I've had a difficult relationship with my mother', Shama says slowly. 'I spent a lot of time away from home trying to work out my feelings about the kind of person she'd want me to be. Now I'm more assertive, she responds to me as a separate person – not belonging to her. When my sister had her baby, she lived with mother and gave in. I'm stronger against my mother. Being a mother myself now I feel very warm to her; up to now it was more a case of "eternally obligated until you die".'

'I can't believe how incredibly demanding being a mother is. There's such a conflict between the person I'd like to be, and bits of my mother I don't like that keep popping out in me. The harder it is, the more I forgive my mother her sins and then feel the baby forgives me mine. I guess it also means I'm more accepting of ambivalence – the beastliness of the child you love', concludes Clarissa, who has been silent.

After the Birth – Shadow Interaction

As these mothers illustrate, further differentiation takes place after the birth when, in their new capacity as parents, relationships with their own mothers and fathers are re-evaluated. A new phase of relating to the infant too begins, as shadowy outlines of fantasy, transposed from pregnancy onto the newly arrived baby begin to recede. Paradoxically, however, as the imaginary baby fades, another baby makes its appearance. Revived by exposure to the raw emotions of their newborn, latent aspects of the parents' own baby selves are rekindled. Suddenly, their adult veneer is in danger of rupturing, as they continually face the crying neediness and physical fragility of a tiny body excreting bodily products from every orifice.

With each developmental phase of their infant, the degree to which each parent has resolved particular infantile conflicts and hungers will determine the degree to which their early emotions flicker into empathic or persecuted responsiveness. Thus we may say that every parent-child couple involves a 'triple shadow interaction': the re-evoked child a parent conjures up having been with her or his own parents; the desired or detested child he or she fantasizes this baby to be in relation to their internal constellation; and the real child whom they are beginning to recognize as an individual. It is when intrapsychic shadows break their bounds, casting depressive or projected darkness of such intensity that it obscures the actual baby that help is required to lift the veil. At this time, psychotherapeutic intervention can shed light on unconscious forces.

An interesting question is how these configurations of a fantasy baby and differing approaches to the pregnancy are reflected in the parent's postnatal relationship with the real infant. And how do we tell? Most care givers hold their babies, feed, change and bathe them, are woken at night by an appeal for comfort, milk, and winding. Yet, how do they differ?

In-depth knowledge of mothers and fathers from pregnancy or even preconception through to early parenthood, suggests that although the sex and personality of each baby inevitably influences caregiving, *antenatal conceptualization of the baby generally primes the parent's orientation.* This means that during pregnancy and in the early days following the birth, based on their own internal models, each woman or man carries in mind an elaborate idea of the kind of parent they wish to be, and a set of beliefs of what babies are like. The scene is set for the post-natal pattern of interaction defined by the same model.

It should be stressed that no one type of relating is advocated; parents can only do what they are comfortable with. Further-more, babies have an uncanny ability to detect fraudulence: people who in adulthood blame their parents for their misery seem more likely to come to terms with an authentic parent, however lacking, than with a deceptive one, however well mean-ing. Pathology lurks in the extremes of each parental orientation, where the adult is unable to recognize the infant and superim-poses a predetermined image or applies such high standards to themselves or to the baby, that disappointment is inevitable. Dif-ficulties may manifest in varying forms of enmeshment or estrangement, possessiveness and/or intrusiveness; from engulf-ing over-involvement, premature or unrealistic expectation, to detachment, chronic disapproval, hostility, violence, and/or over-regimentation.

The Facilitator

The Facilitator approaches motherhood as a long-awaited, deeply gratifying experience. Drawing her baby to her breast immediately after the birth – sometimes even before the cord is cut – she is determined not to be separated from the infant whom she feels is still part of her and symbiotically attached: birth is a reunion with a beloved.

The Facilitator believes that biological synchrony during preg-nancy and prenatal communion has established a special under-standing between them. In her empathic state of heightened sensitivity, the Facilitator feels strongly that she alone has the intuitive capacity to interpret the baby's needs: 'We are so close, I can feel inside myself what she needs.' Since no one can take her place, the baby is totally reliant upon her continuous presence. Jealously guarding the bubble of exclusive intimacy in which she is enveloped with the dependent baby, the Facilitator intends to dedicate herself fully to deciphering and meeting her newborn's needs spontaneously and immediately.

Following the baby's guide, the Facilitator offers her breast unrestrictedly, feeds on demand for as long as the baby wishes to suck day and night (weaning usually occurs between one and two years, unless instigated by the infant). As every sound is deemed an appeal, she has to maintain constant vigilance at all times. She keeps the baby close, in her arms or a body-sling most of the day, and in her room or bed at night. The couple's sexual activity may be postponed for some months as the infant continues to wake, often several times a night. Close proximity during the night alerts the mother to any little sound from her baby, and, conversely, the smell of her milk and the sound of her stirring may penetrate the baby's sleep. Indeed, sleep may be experienced as a separation by the mother, who longs to re-establish their prenatal fusion. Yearning to recapture this illusion of perfect, primal oneness, the Facilitator often denies any hint of ambivalence, idealizing her gratified baby, and herself as bountiful mother, maintaining an invisible umbilicus in the emotional, placental processing.

The Regulator

By contrast, the Regulator regards maternal devotion as an over-rated myth, propagated by society to keep mothers at home. She is determined to avoid becoming submerged in domesticity by returning to her 'real' life as soon as possible. Taking time to recuperate after the birth, she does not mind separating from the new baby, who at first seems a stranger she will gradually come to know.

Unlike the Facilitator, who aims to gratify her baby's every wish, the Regulator believes the caregiver's basic task is to socialize the presocial (or asocial) baby, regularizing his or her impulses in preparation for the demands of the world at large. She maintains it is wrong to give her child a false sense of herself as the exclusive source of comfort: the model she presents is of a variety of caring people. In her view, mothering is not inborn but an acquired skill that can be learned.

Since she believes the newborn does not differentiate between carers, the Regulator mother introduces co-carers early on, once she has established optimal regularity. To this end she sets up a *routine*, which ensures predictability in the shapeless and potentially bewildering situation, and provides mother and baby with a sense of security. She feeds the baby at regular intervals, for a set time per feed; gives supplementary bottles if breastfeeding to enable other caregivers to feed; and intends to begin weaning with the introduction of solids. Following a schedule enables the Regulator and other carers to provide continuity and to be consistent in determining the baby's needs, while distinguishing between what she deems 'legitimate' crying and 'fussing':

> 'I knew it couldn't be hunger or wind because it was only two hours since the last feed. He'd been changed before being put down for his nap, and wasn't due to wake for another half hour. There were no pins in his nappy. When I peeped in he was still covered with his blanket and wasn't cold, so I let him bawl, which he did for a while, then tired himself out and went back to sleep.'

The routine also provides the mother with a degree of freedom. Once her baby becomes regularized to the regime, proximity is no longer imperative. She or he can be left in containers – carry-cot, bouncy-chair or pram – by day, and sleeps in his/her own bedroom, where the baby reportedly sleeps through the night from an early age, which is measured in weeks rather than months.

While the Facilitator adapts herself to her baby, the Regulator expects the baby to adapt to the household routine.

The Reciprocator

Although Reciprocators appear to occupy an intermediate position between Facilitators and Regulators, and do indeed engage in both types of behaviour, they too have a philosophy of baby care. From the first, Reciprocators tend to perceive the child as a potentially whole and multifaceted person with whom they can interact. As the infant is seen to occupy different states of alertness which determine the level of interaction, there is constant *negotiation* rather than a pattern of either facilitation or regulation.

Rather than seeing the new baby as social but symbiotically merged with and dependent upon the mother like the Facilitator, or as separate and in need of socialization like the Regulator, the

Reciprocator sees the newborn as a separate, outgoing, sociable person capable of forming relationships and of making demands. Since the infant is regarded as sharing similar emotions to the parents, albeit at a different level of sophistication, the Reciprocator parent feels she or he can learn to understand the baby, and can come to be understood:

> 'It's wonderful to have someone who can look at me and recognize me and accept me just as I am', says the mother of three-week-old Alice. 'We're all discovering new worlds – we're getting to know her as a person and she's teaching us about ourselves as parents. I'm learning her different cries, but sometimes we have hitches in communicating. She's not a helpless creature – she also makes decisions and decides how she wants to be. Often she's quite alert and not upset, just watching the world and taking things in, and responding. She loves people, but if I keep her waiting for a feed because I'm busy, she can get quite angry and impatient with me. I've learned that when she's so hungry she can't grasp the nipple properly and hits it instead of sucking. She also senses my tension with my cracked nipple, but if I warn her first, she's quite gentle, and doesn't seem frustrated if I explain why I'm being slow.'

Reciprocators believe in reciprocal companionship and reciprocal respect. They feel the baby's needs are entitled to full consideration, but, by the same token, so are everybody else's in the family, including the parents'. Special concessions are made to the infant's inability to wait, and his or her limitations in communicating and understanding language, or holding on to a memory for very long. However, this does not mean always putting the baby's needs first, nor adapting family life entirely to the baby's rhythms, nor getting the baby to adapt to their own. Adjustments are continually being made, as daily routines and activities are reassessed according to the baby's mood, development, and changing needs, and the constant fluctuations of the general household and the caregivers' need for work or space.

Clearly, maintaining a high degree of flexibility and the complex juggling of everyone's needs is a difficult proposition. In some ways it is much simpler to stick to a regular routine, or to devote all one's efforts to meeting the baby's needs first and foremost. And indeed, Reciprocators often find themselves unable to keep everyone equally in mind. Nevertheless, as with all parenting, the capacity to recognize mistakes and reflect about potential causes and remedies helps them return to their preferred course.

Relating the Two Models

If we now re-examine the placental paradigm in light of this descriptive model, we can see in the table below that each maternal position is based on a particular combination of internal representations of herself and the baby.

Beliefs Underpinning Parental Orientation

	Facilitator	Reciprocator	Regulator
Mode	mother adapts	negotiation	baby adapts
Assumptions	baby knows best	neither knows, both can find out	mother/expert knows
Basis	identification	inter-subjectivity	detachment
Neonate	symbiotic, sociable	different levels of alertness	non-discriminating, asocial, pre-social
Maternal task	processing	interaction	socialization
Goal	dependence → mature dependence	lifelong inter-dependence	dependence → independence
Unconscious attribution	baby is ideal self (fear of hating)	baby is a person (acceptance of ambivalence)	baby represents repudiated self (fear of loving)

Unconscious Identifications

Clearly, the experience of the early postnatal weeks differs a great deal for each mother, who in turn creates a unique environment for her newborns. How can we explain the experiential differences that underpin maternal orientations? Donald Winnicott described a state of heightened sensitivity he called primary maternal preoccupation, in which an 'aspect of the mother's personality takes over temporarily' based on her capacity for identification with the baby. For the Facilitator, this condition seems to begin in early pregnancy, and is based on an unconscious identification of her idealized baby self with the fantasized baby. The imaginary baby can be conceptualized as a flawless *ideal self* or a glorified ideal of *mother-baby fusion*. Narcissistic identification with both mother and baby is transmuted postnatally into empathic gratification of the baby as an extension of the self. This serves the dual purpose of vicarious self-compensation and reparation to the mother's own mother.

However, as we have seen, not all mothers have a positive view of themselves, or a pleasant emotional experience of the baby. To some, already during pregnancy the fetus feels exploitative, and the fantasy baby may represent not cherished but repudiated aspects of the self: a dependent, weak, greedy, or sadistic denigrated baby self. Since what are internalized are relationships rather than individuals, this image of a baby self is usually coupled with a care giver seen as overrated, critical, depriving, or drained. For the Regulator, a defensive compromise could reside in avoiding conflict over the maternal role itself, which may be denigrated, or seem unachievable in view of her own self-depreciation in contrast to her own over-estimated mother. Strategies may involve rebellion ('I'll never be a dormat like my mother!'); circumvention ('What babies really need is lots of relationships'); abrogation of responsibility ('The nanny does what's necessary'); or safeguarding her own competence ('It depresses me trying to be what I'm not. I'm no good at most of this mothering stuff, so I do what I *am* good at.').

The crux of the matter is that a Facilitator is afraid of hating; many a Regulator is afraid of loving. In her idealization, a Facilitator unconsciously expresses fear of her own ambivalence, needing to preserve the myth of unconditional, boundless, munificent mother love, and unable to contemplate her own neediness; the Regulator avoids the trap of falling in love and being sucked into identification with the baby or with her mother. A woman who feels that her own love has been rejected, or even treated as dangerous by early caregivers and/or adult lovers, may wish to protect the baby from the powerful intensity of her feelings by keeping her emotional distance, or controlling her passion by setting limits through the routine.

For the Facilitator, loss of enriching pregnancy is redeemed by reflected glory, as she identifies herself with the perfect infant she has produced and vicariously gratifies her own needs by cosetting the baby during the 'honeymoon' following the birth. Her defensive idealization, however, is maintained at a cost, namely by:

- denial of imperfections of motherhood and baby;
- disavowal of underlying feelings of envy, rivalry, irritation, depression, and aggression;
- altruistic surrender and suspension of personal needs and non-maternal adult interests;
- fostering of an illusion to undo and negate separateness;
- manic reparation to deny guilt and avoid frustration.

For the Regulator, emotionally impoverishing pregnancy not only depleted her of her familiar identity, but postnatally she fears competition with the greedy baby over her own meagre resources, which are without possibility of replenishment. She may also feel in competition with her mother, who is felt to have deprived her in infancy, or to have been so efficient that she, the new mother, cannot hope to compete. Unconsciously, the baby represents a threat of exposure on four counts:

- having been inside her, the infant is seen to be disparaging or critical and can lay bare her hidden badness;
- the baby, who is her product, not only reveals her poor workmanship, but by unseemly behaviour can show her up as an incompetent mother;
- exposure to the raw needs and primitive emotions of the dependent newborn may evoke infantile experiences, which re-awaken early deficits and vulnerability, decentering her hard-earned adult competence.
- the baby's defencelessness increases the mother's temptation to dominate it – and the aspect of herself the baby represents – thereby raising her fears of losing control in an effort to make the 'naughty' baby 'good'.

Thus for the Regulator every cry can be deemed a criticism or exposure, an insatiable demand for more than she can offer, and emotional blackmail with a ransom beyond her means. Projecting her internal objects on to the baby, she dreads not only the judgmental baby's sadistic attacks, but her own retaliatory ones: the danger that she herself could become the dangerous mother, or be engulfed by the dangerous baby. We can see why for the Regulator these early weeks bring not primary maternal preoccupation but a state I call *primary maternal persecution*.

Many Regulators safeguard against the multiple perils of early motherhood by various forms of dissociation:

- forgoing vicarious gratification, whereby regression and breakthrough of her neediness are avoided;
- defence mechanisms, which by splitting and negating fantasy protect her from recognition of unconscious identifications;
- fortification of control and rigidification of defences, thereby curtailing emotional involvement;
- instigation of a routine, eliminating the need for empathic responsiveness; minimizing dangers of neglect or over-indulgence, and the thrust of envying the baby's care;
- shared care, which safeguards her resources, reducing the degree of exposure. This diffuses persecutory anxiety of projected and retaliatory hostility, and avoids possessiveness, assuaging the guilt of usurping her internal mother.

The Reciprocator, who is aware of an ambivalent mixture, appears to be able to accept both her own and the baby's good and bad aspects: 'My baby is wonderful and I love her dearly, but when she wakes me for the umpteenth time I could strangle her.' This tolerance is related to co-existence of various senses of self – physical, social, and intrapsychic, preverbal and speeched – and feeling at ease with both masculine and feminine identifications, experienced simultaneously. The capacity to encompass full richness of the personality without excessively hiving sections off also enables the Reciprocator to experience infantile needs without threat or secret craving, and indulge them without relinquishing adulthood.

Inter-Relationships with Partners

Mothers and babies do not exist in a vacuum; even during pregnancy a woman's orientation is guided by external as well as internal reality. In the early postnatal period, a Facilitator mother cannot dedicate herself to facilitating her baby devotedly unless someone is providing for her and taking prime responsibility for shopping, ferrying other children around, and helping with household chores. Likewise, a Regulator may long for adult company and the opportunity to exercise her competence, but if unemployed she may find herself isolated with her baby, particularly if she lacks the means to hire someone to care for the child.

Increasingly, many mothers live alone, either through choice or circumstance. Others live with a male partner who is not the baby's father. Some live in lesbian couples, and may be facing social prejudice or legal difficulties in addition to the hardships of early parenting, role allocation, and adjustments within the partnership. A cohabiting partner does not necessarily make things easier, especially if their views on babycare do not tally.

Using the same model – and always remembering that in reality there are few pure types – we may speak of the partner as a Facilitator, Reciprocator or Regulator in their own right.

However, another dimension enters into partnering. Although biology restricts childbearing to females, society, which has hitherto automatically allocated primary care to women, is beginning to change. As yet, the dimension of choice that exists regarding which partner carries the baby in some lesbian couples is absent in heterosexual couples, where it is still the woman who bears the baby. However, men are now granted previously absent socially sanctioned choices in relation to childcare. We may therefore speak of a spectrum of Participator partners, who wish to participate as much as possible in looking after the baby, and Renouncer partners, who renounce their nurturing capacities.

The Participator

A Participator may feel elated when following the long ordeal of pregnancy at one remove, and excruciatingly helpless during the experience of watching the exciting birth, at which point he or she can finally greet the baby directly. If during pregnancy unconscious identification with the fetus has granted vicarious re-entry to the maternal womb, parenthood allows the Participator symbolic repossession of infancy.

Drawing on maternal aspects rooted in early identification with the nurturing mother, whom he or she may try to emulate or surpass, the partner cradles and croons, strokes and caresses the newborn and takes over most of the babycare, if partnered with a Regulator. If the mother is a Facilitator, respective desires for exclusivity may clash: 'I yearn to be everything to my son, but she has the milk and she was there first', says a Participator father poignantly. If neither parent concedes their desire for exclusivity, they may compete in their respective needs to be the best nurturer ('Who do you love best, baby – Mummy or Daddy?'). Other solutions may consist of a compromise where primary care giving is shared: 'At first she seemed to take over and I felt left out. But I realized we couldn't be the same – we're different, and the baby sees us differently too. I absolutely adore him and can do most things for him except breastfeed, so we share but each do things in our own way.' Or else the partner mothers the mother so she can mother the baby.

The Renouncer

By contrast, the Renouncer partner feels quite clear about the division of labour, renouncing feminine aspects of his early identification: 'I'm sure I will be close to my son when he's one or two. I know it's old-fashioned, but just now I'm proud to be looking after my family, protecting them and being the breadwinner.' A Facilitator mother may rejoice in this traditional arrangement, which gives her the exclusive care of the baby, provided the Renouncer partner supports her full-time mothering. In this traditional household, mother and baby form the primary unit, if the partner can tolerate or even prefers being on the emotional sidelines. However, some may find the sight of their women feeding or cosseting the baby disturbing, and occasionally a mother may feel compelled to change her babycare practices to accommodate her partner's sensitivities: 'He treated my breastfeeding as if I was committing incest or adultery. I've had to give up nightfeeding altogether and just feed during the day when he's not around. It feels furtive.'

Conversely, a Regulator mother may want her Renouncer partner to relieve her of some childcare duties, or at least to endorse her decision to resume her old life of work or social activities, which may necessitate paying for a childminder. Their compromise solution might be shared baby care, or in a dual-career family, both partners leaving it to another care giver. In their case, there may be a clearcut division not between genders but between generations – with the couple as the primary emotional unit. Sexuality is usually resumed in such couples earlier than in an undisturbed Facilitator-Renouncer one.

Postnatal Distress

Many women experience the minor mood fluctuations associated with the transient state of tearfulness called 'maternity blues', which passes within a week or two after the birth. However, more persistent postnatal depression is fairly prevalent. This may take the form of mild distress, which is suffered by almost half of all mothers at some time before their child is two, and is accompanied by tearfulness, anxiety, and irritability. Severe depression, suffered by up to one-quarter of all new mothers, includes symptoms of self-neglect; suicidal tendencies; sleep, libido, and appetite disorders; and feelings of profound self-depreciation, helplessness, self-loathing, inadequacy, and despair.

In classical studies, contributing factors have been found to relate to early emotional deprivation, poor social support, marital difficulties, lack of employment, and ambivalence about the pregnancy.

In my own studies, I have found that precipitating factors of postnatal depression differ according to each woman's maternal orientation: thus, lack of employment might distress a Regulator, but the converse is true for a Facilitator. We can also be more specific about the nature of marital difficulties: a mismatch of parental orientations can constitute a precipitating factor to postnatal distress. For instance, sometimes a traditional Renouncer, on the basis of his own internalized model of parenting, insists that his wife be a housebound mother. While suiting a Facilitator, if a woman is a Regulator at heart, this curtailment of her independence will be distressing, especially if she is denied the adult company she craves, and feels unable to reinstate her previous identity when stuck at home with a demanding baby. Continuous exposure to the infant may seem threatening and depleting, and if she feels the baby to be judgmental, she may experience primary maternal persecution, particularly if she is unable to find time for herself, or is made to feel guilty and reproached for wanting to leave her child.

Bipolar Conflict

Distress may result not only from an external imposition, but from an internal mismatch. A woman's self-esteem may be jeopardized as she feels herself torn between the orientation she has anticipated prenatally, and the materialization of her capacities as a mother:

> 'I feel I'm not allowed to be a real person. I'm supposed to be totally devoted, but when I'm with him I'm always wishing I was somewhere else, or that he'd go to sleep and not need me. It's unbearable for me because all the things I depend on to feel my usual self – like reading and sleeping and keeping myself looking trim and well-dressed – are incompatible with being a full-time mother. I'm trying to do things right, and am afraid that if I deviate at all from our routine all hell will break loose. Ever since his excruciating birth I haven't had the space to recuperate and pull myself together and feel good about myself as a person, and I'm turning out to be such a terrible mother.'

The above quote is from a depressed woman in therapy. Her Regulator internal mother criticizes her constantly for not being tough enough; her Facilitator conscience pricks her for not being devoted enough, while in her depression, she cannot regain her sense of self or find a way to meet her own, as well as the baby's, needs for a 'good start'.

Such bipolar conflicts – where a mother is torn between Facilitator and Regulator extremes within herself – (sometimes internally represented by her two parents) can be extremely painful and distressing. She may feel caught between a desire to provide 'unlimited, immediate and everlasting gratification' (as Melanie Klein, in 1952 described the ideal 'inexhaustible breast') and the ravaging fears of her own badness, and/or the baby's greed or judgement. She may feel like this woman:

> 'I get such sinister feelings when I'm breastfeeding in my mother's presence, or even just think of her. My milk turns to poison, and when he cries or vomits I feel accused and I hear her voice inside my ear saying, "You're doing it wrong". I so want to get it right, but I don't want to follow *her* rulebook approach. But when I follow the baby, I hear her snarling,

"Stop feeding him so much". Whichever way I turn, I can't win', says a mother who cannot tolerate her baby's crying without her own tears flowing.

To mother generously, a mother needs to feel mothered. The absence of a loving mother or partner to support her in reality, or to enrich her from within, can make a woman veer from trying to live up to an idealized idea of herself as the perfect mother she never had, to being a deprived daughter who feels a gap instead of maternal resources. A mother in therapy says of her postnatal depression many years earlier:

'When my baby didn't smile, I felt he was witholding from me. On the other hand, sometimes I resented him clinging to me and refusing to go to others. He just wanted *me* all the time. I felt smothered by more demands than I was capable of responding to. I needed someone to share it, and to give me as I was giving. Other people had their mothers, but my mother was dead, and my husband didn't really understand. I felt I was getting nothing good from anybody.'

Therapy, providing a woman with care and access to a benevolent internal mother, helps a troubled woman to help herself. The Facilitator mother's close identification with her baby offers a vicarious experience of being mothered herself; however, the Regulator who feels in competition with her infant over scarce resources may be indignant about demands made upon her, or even envy the care she herself provides (envy of her own breast).

A babyminder who grants the mother time out can serve a dual purpose of protecting the mother from the experience of the infant's ascribed criticism ('When I feed her, she looks daggers at me – but I can't help it if my milk is thin'); and providing time away which reduces the risk of emotional 'contamination' (being sucked back into old dependencies) and allows her the opportunity to replenish her adult resources. 'Work is my sanity', says one depressed Regulator. 'When I'm stuck at home with the screeching baby, I feel I'm going crazy and don't know who I am anymore, or what he wants from me or how long I can stand his clinging dependence without throwing him out of the window.' If a Regulator has doubts about her maternal qualities, shared care not only shelters the baby from her constant influence, but gives her an alibi against future blame of being the sole cause of the child's illbeing. A Regulator mother who is intent on mitigating her own 'bad' forces and persecutory internal presences, may employ a Facilitator caregiver to provide positive ones she feels she lacks.

Likewise, a Facilitator may suffer depression postnatally, precipitated not by enforced *togetherness*, but by enforced *separation*. If she has had to leave her baby before she feels ready to do so due to economic pressures, preterm birth, medical problems, or social demands, not only will she feel she has betrayed her own standards of perfection, but fears she may have caused her baby irrevocable emotional harm. Equally, if the birth or early months have not been trouble-free, the Facilitator may have difficulty seeing herself as the ideal, generous, good mother, feeling she has become a bad or injurious mother to her vulnerable, innocent and trusting baby, and inflicting long-lasting damage: 'The birth was so bloody awful, I felt I'd betrayed his trust, and our relationship was spoilt before it even began.'

Such relationships may become complicated by the Facilitator mother desperately trying to assuage her guilt to compensate for past imperfections. In fact, rather than mothering, she begins to practise 'psychotherapy' with her child. The same events may colour the early days differently for a Regulator, with a sense of having had something 'bloody awful' inflicted upon *her*. Working it through, the Reciprocator will enable such a 'bloody awful' start to be absorbed into their mutual history.

Looked at in terms of the placental paradigm, the Facilitator, who has started with a view of herself as a good mother to a good baby, finds she has inadvertently become bad, and is anguished by her inability to right all of the wrongs, as a postnatally depressed, would-be Facilitator says:

'When Jason cries it tears me apart deep inside because I can't give him what he really wants. My placenta wasn't good enough to nourish him until term, and he was born early, before his liver could cope, so he was jaundiced; I felt I'd ruined him. I wanted to give him everything to make up for it, and wept such bitter tears over his first bottle after my milk dried up. How can I ever make it up to him?'

Underlying expectations will predispose mothers of different orientations to vulnerability at specific periods of the baby's development. Thus an extreme Facilitator who has a profound inability to give up an illusory state of emotional fusion with the baby after the initial months, will feel endangered by the growing infant's healthy need to differentiate and separate. Distressed, the mother may unconsciously resort to increasingly desperate attempts to remain the sole source of succour. She may intrusively try to control the baby's thoughts and feelings, pre-empting self-expression. False-self placatory smiling, and the baby's reassurance that the mother is indeed a perfect provider, are often evidence of a prohibition on crying, unconsciously registered by the extreme Facilitator as an accusation about her insufficiency or an individualizing complaint. The mother may even resent his or her self-contained musing and gazing round during feeding, and particularly thumb-sucking, as indications of self-sufficiency. She may actually step up feeding at this point, actively interpreting every communication as a desire for her breast, jealous of other intimates, treating even sleep as a betrayal of their closeness.

Conversely, a Regulator might rejoice in signs of the baby's increasing independence. An extreme Regulator, however, might foster these prematurely. Resenting their interdependency, she may wean the baby abruptly, often having experienced breast-feeding as unpleasantly cannibalistic. She too may forbid crying as being accusatory or critical of her maternal abilities, glad to be released from mothering by a substitute caregiver or work. If she is unable to get away, and the baby is invested with characteristics of negative internal figures such as her own mother or father, she may assign the baby a parental role, feeling trapped with a demanding, nagging, or neglectful carer who does not fulfil her expectations. As with a Facilitator's baby, who is ascribed adoration duties, the Regulator's may develop an acute awareness of the mother's or father's need to be looked after, at times inhibiting or forgoing their own needs for nurturing.

When unconsciously regarded as an extension of herself, the Regulator's baby can feel particularly persecuting. Experiencing her inner badness shown up by the unruly child – who displays her ineffectiveness by crying inconsolably, and parades her internal badness by picking its nose or farting – she may resort to physical means to quell the baby's badness and make it good.

The period from about six to twelve months is usually a rewarding one for many Regulators, who find the increasingly active and interesting baby's affectionate recognition of them touching. However, with rapid crawling and upright mobility the baby becomes dangerously unpredictable once more, needing constant surveillance. By contrast, when the newly mobile *rapprochement*-stage toddler alternates independence with a clingy need for reassurance, the Facilitator mother may feel she has had a reprieve, and has her baby back.

In general, mothers who have had definite expectations may become disappointed and severely distressed by a baby who fails to live up to their parental hopes or postnatal symbolic representations. Reciprocators, who await the unfolding of the baby's personal characteristics, are protected by a relative lack of expectations. However, a modicum of depression is an inevitable part of the Reciprocator's recognition of ambivalence.

In sum, I am proposing that although it takes many forms, *postnatal distress is a function of interpersonal, physical, economic or socio-cultural factors conspiring to prevent each mother from fulfilling her own specific expectations of motherhood.* Precipitating factors differ for Facilitator and Regulator mothering.

The Power of the Past

A parent's baby-care orientations are rooted in their own babyhood. Expectations and conscious beliefs about newborns as being benign or wild, symbiotically merged, or undiscriminating, and about themselves as parents, draw on multiple unconscious configurations of themselves as babies, and reactivated conflicts relating to the nurturing they imagine they received. The more complex and fluid these mental constructs are, the less rigid the parental stance. There is no simple linear trajectory by which a parent follows the practice of their own parent. Rather, mothers' and fathers' parenting may identify with, or may be a reaction-formation (doing the opposite) against, or operates in competition with, their current view of internal parents and experiences of being parented. We have each imbibed unconscious preoccupations of our care givers alongside their conscious expectations. These may come into play and are repeated generation after generation, as each parent in turn is spurred on by internal driving forces.

A Facilitator, for example, might crave the idealized infancy she believes she had by emulating her glorified mother. Conversely, she may feel compelled to use mother/baby fusion to make reparation to her mother for her own real or imagined attacks. Or she may omnipotently wish to outdo her mother, compensating for infantile deficiencies; or, by being different hopes vicariously to provide the perfect experience of which she feels deprived. Likewise, a Regulator might feel she is doing as she was done by, using scheduled feeding to curb her own projected greed; alternatively, she may try providing her baby with a security and predictability she never had. Others may refuse to become identified with a denigrated mother ('I'll never be like her'), or avoid engagement in devalued motherhood ('It's a ploy to keep women domesticated'). Through projective identification, both Facilitators and Regulators invest split-off aspects of their self-representations into their unconscious representation of the baby. The former can then indulge in vicarious gratification but must remain connected; the latter experiences persecutory anxiety unless protected by detachment.

What we, external observers, see in parent-baby interactions, are the loving gestures, compromise formations, and defensive measures employed by mothers and fathers in the face of the highly arousing, primitive emotions of their infant, and their own internal infant selves. Given their individual psychological histories and degree of emotional preoccupation with the past, each parent will be affected differently by the yelling/smiling infant in their care, and at different developmental stages respond more or less intensely to the demands and tribulations of parenthood as they personally experience it.

Parental orientation pivots on a complex, swirling mixture of unconscious configurations of the baby, selectively recalled early memories composed of nebulous images, and salient fragments of pre-ideational sensory-semiotic experience as well as modified fantasies. All these determine and are determined by the person's present emotional state. In addition, these configurations are not only coloured by present and past emotions, but also incorporate the original caregiver's own unconscious representations – the 'ghostly' presences transmitted by the parent, intuited and experienced by the son or daughter, and unconsciously handed on through the generations. These 'ghosts in the nursery', as Selma

Fraiberg termed them, do not tally with that caregiver's actual behaviour: 'When my baby cries at night, my heart pounds and I feel this strange sense of anxiety, a real fear of death. Although she never admitted it, I think I've always known my mother was gripped by panic under all that false calm.' Other parents may have endeavoured to follow child-care practices recommended at the time, which were at variance with personal orientation: 'My grandmother told me she would sit with tears rolling down her cheeks as she watched the clock until the next decreed four-hourly scheduled feeding.'

The Next Time Round

As noted, a woman who has been pregnant before will engage with subsequent pregnancies in a different way from her first. If she has had a miscarriage, the loss of trust will have sensitized her to the possibility of things going wrong; an abortion may haunt her in a way it hasn't before, as the weeks roll by until this pregnancy is 'new' rather than a re-experience of the previous one.

If she has had a child, almost from the beginning she will be awaiting a *baby*, a person who is already forming within her. Aware of the personalities and characteristics of her other children, and the way these have unfolded at each phase, it is easier for her to visualize the new baby. Paradoxically, she may also be aware of how different he or she may be.

Looking back at their previous experience, women who found it difficult to relate to the preverbal infant can with hindsight now recognize how much is grasped and built upon, even at those early stages. Understanding how sensitive and observant the baby is from the first, and that he or she is acting on healthy needs rather than driven by whims or greedy cravings, makes it easier for the mother to relate to her next child. Even in early pregnancy she will have a stronger sense of the baby as an individual, and a belief in his or her future relationship to her as a special person – rather than a placenta or breast to be made use of.

In a subsequent wanted pregnancy, recognizing her importance for the fetus will necessitate having to protect the baby's birthrights, as well as safeguarding everyone's needs for emotional and practical support, and personal space.

I shall illustrate this complex emotional juggling with a vignette from a woman I have been seeing weekly throughout her first pregnancy and her daughter Alice's babyhood.

In the preceding two sessions, she has complained of nausea and hypersensitive tearfulness – 'Raw, as if one's skin's removed' – suspecting pregnancy, although she has not had a period since conceiving Alice. Here she is telling me, in thirteen-month-old Alice's presence, that it has been confirmed that she is indeed expecting another baby:

> 'I am thrilled to be pregnant. I want babies quite close in age', says Alice's mother, as her daughter picks up a little plastic 'playperson' and kisses its head saying, 'Dadda'.
>
> 'Alice is a bit clingy. She hates it when I vomit – it's quite frightening for her.' Alice now has a plastic doll in her mouth and is knocking it with the other one, clearly clowning and trying to divert her mother's attention while seemingly responding to her words.
>
> 'I had the eight-week scan this week. We got a photograph for David. Alice sat near my knees and saw the little blob on the screen – very exciting, nice to have confirmation, although with this nausea I didn't need it. The first time round, pregnancy was such a mystery, and I couldn't connect it with having something at the end of it all.'
>
> Alice is now engrossed in the book her mother is adeptly showing her while talking to me, and gleefully making roaring sounds to a picture of a lion. She looks up as her mother completes her sentence, grinning at her. Her mother responds by grimacing and roaring, too.
>
> 'Although I feel very emotional,' she muses momentarily, holding Alice's face in her hands and peering closely at her, 'I can't quite work out this feeling of detachment – there is a strange sense of a secret place in which the baby is growing.' Alice gets down off her knee.
>
> I comment on a possible sense of disloyalty at holding someone else in mind in addition to Alice. 'I desperately needed space last week and time to myself to think about it.'
>
> Alice, who has been standing in the toy basket sucking her thumb, now lifts her arms to be taken back on to her mother's lap. She's held there securely and given a box of raisins. 'I suppose every mother goes through this with each baby, and

they seem to survive', she comments as Alice deftly eats her raisins one by one.

'Last time I felt unable to do anything or keep anything down. When I wasn't sure about the pregnancy, and gave David a hard time. I was angry with him it was hard to visualize our ongoing relationship, let alone a baby. It just seemed like a trap of an endless round of chronic nausea and vomiting, which I resented like mad. Now I feel just as sick, but I know what it's about. I trust my body, and remembering how much better it eventually got last time, I can wait. Meanwhile, David is very sympathetic and in love with me, but all my deep emotional senses are heightened and David feels I'm slipping away a bit. I do feel out of tune – he's working hard and distracted and I'm feeling distant . . . Not resentful, but separate.'

Alice has got down and is examining the contents of her mother's handbag as she speaks, leaning over to feed her mother a raisin. 'She's been waking a lot during the last three nights. David brings her back to our bed – He does, doesn't he? And in the mornings, with this nausea, I just collapse on to the settee, which frustrates Alice. It must be confusing for her to see me behaving differently.'

Alice has seated herself on a little rug, legs outstretched. She takes the last few raisins out of the box then puts the last two back again. 'She's a delight, but there's been a change, and she seems to sense the change in me, and would cry if I left the room.' Alice begins looking for a lost raisin saying, 'Gone'. Her mother finds it under the couch and hands it to her, 'Here it is'. Once again Alice seems to reflect a tacit awareness of the content of our conversation. Equally, although involved in her own thoughts, Alice's mother is remarkably attuned and intuitively responsive to the variations in her daughter's moods.

'She's a real chatterbox in her own language. She's not as demanding on my body as she used to be, and not really breast-feeding, although she takes a suck now and then, just to make sure they're still there. Don't you?' Alice grins, putting head down on the floor, looking across at me upside down through her legs, clutching her now empty little box. Then she cries briefly as she steps on a toy, and her mother lifts and cuddles her while Alice sucks her thumb. As she recovers and struggles down again, her mother says, 'We seem to have lost any routine. I can't predict when, if at all, I'll find time for myself or get some work done. But she's such good fun at the moment, entertaining – and inventive.'

Here is the same mother nine months later, in my consulting room suckling her six-week-old baby daughter, Wendy:

'I feel so happy watching them together. Alice is so sweet with her, although she does try to sit on her, or put her finger in her mouth, or get Wendy to open her eyes. In some ways it's much more than twice-times-one having two children. There's so little time to just watch Wendy as I did Alice. It's more than double the work, and at times I feel quite isolated and lonely. We just collapse at 10.30, too exhausted to appreciate each other's company. I really have to remind myself I'm not hard done by, because it's so easy to feel unsupported, although David does as much as he possibly can. My body is never my own – sometimes I feel mauled by each in turn.'

Intrapsychic and Socio-Cultural Influences

Parental orientations may change with the next baby. Throughout our lives, not only do our external relationships vary, but different versions of internal figures alter and diversify with our emotional experience. In general, availability of loving memories, loveable aspects of ourselves, and the sense of love-ability bestowed by a responsive internal caring figure, fluctuate at different times, affected by life events and affecting our interpretation of them.

Changes in parental orientation reflect changes within the inner world. Emotional growth and resolution of conflicts within the person's psyche are very much influenced by the experience of rearing the previous baby. Birth and becoming a parent are major life events.

Parental orientation is influenced by a multitude of socio-economic and interpersonal variables: the composition of the household, whether there is a caring partner, and his or her parental orientation. The age and number of other children (it appears that more first-time mothers are Regulators); the age-gaps between them (it is difficult to facilitate a second child close in age to the first); the parent's age, interests, career status, and expectations; and the degree of social and material support available. In my view, the most important determinants are intrapsychic.

Over my years of specialization, the model has been gradually elaborated through clinical work with individuals, and couples, and mother-child observations, which have been augmented by surveys of pre- and postnatal parental attitudes. When I first published the model in 1983, maternal conceptualization and practice appeared polarized between the Facilitator and Regulator orientations, with an intermediate group. In subsequent work, the middle group grew in proportion, and has taken on a definite character. I attribute this change partly to my increased understanding, and partly to an increasing popular interest and promotion by the media of information on the capacities of newborn babies that underpin the Reciprocator orientation.

Although Facilitator- and Regulator-type stances had been around for many years, they had been masked by social pressures towards wholesale adherence to popular childcare fashions, such as the regulatory era of Truby King, or the permissive one of Dr Spock. In recent years, greater freedom of reproductive choice for women has followed in the wake of rapid political and socio-economic changes, including wartime establishment of daycare nurseries and postwar self-help facilities, the advent of the contraceptive pill and legal access to abortions, and increasing affiliation of women in a more variegated labour force. Simultaneously, ideological enforcement of Facilitator and Regulator orientations have come from popularized psychoanalytic ideas on child-rearing, and from the women's movement.

On the one hand, John Bowlby's early ideas were widely publicized following the second world war, focusing on monotrophic attachment and the adverse effects of maternal separation (this was misinterpreted as advocating night and day, seven days a week, 365 days a year devotion), and Donald Winnicott's broadcasts to parents, resonated with Facilitators, and endorsed Renouncer-type traditional paternity, as have some family therapists. On the other hand, Betty Friedan's explosive exposure of the *Feminine Mystique* and explorations of sexual politics, decrease in family size, demands for equal work opportunities, and daycare facilities influenced and ratified would-be Regulators.

Concurrently, the resurgence of female participation in the public sphere, coupled with demands for shared childcare, has enabled male Participators to become domestically involved in childrearing, inviting them to share in antenatal care, birth, and raising their babies. Class, age, and sexist stratification have been challenged with consequent tendencies towards unisex equalization. Conversely, in recent years, gender polarization and the separatist position of many feminists has been modified to focus on similarities between the sexes and studying differences within gender groups.

My overview, therefore, is that on a societal level, received ideas and accepted concepts of morality which had been questioned and liberated in the mid-1960s, then underwent a further sea-change from an emphasis on personal fulfilment in the mid-1970s to an ethic of greater reciprocal responsibility in the late 1980s and wider transcultural social liability in the 1990s. I believe it is this change that is reflected in the increasing proportion of the groups of parents I call Reciprocators. They flourish in an ideological climate of personal choice yet global responsibility, which advocates individuation but recognizes accountability of people to each other, to their own community and beyond, to their society and worldwide issues. These preoccupations are reflected in media and educational popularization of such topics as research findings on the capacities of newborn infants and fetuses, heightened awareness of the psychosocial effects of racism, sexism, ageism, and legal redefinitions of entitlement (for example, fetal rights and children as competent witnesses, coerced marital-coition redefined as rape), public exposure of leadership failures and recognition of the need for global ecological policies on environmental protection, etc. People who engage in reciprocal parenting struggle daily with the paradoxical dilemma of intersubjectivity: granting rights to one member of the carer-baby tandem means the other is entitled too.

Increased liberalization of parental roles and child care practices offers a greater variety of choices to the Western mother and father. These open new opportunities for expressive relationships in accordance with each person's psychic reality, rather than the dictates of sociocultural expectations. It is a sobering thought that the positive freedom thus granted is counterbalanced by the risk of its abuse, when internal fantasy is translated into action. Hence the importance of liberating therapy from its stigma and from its elitist image, and investing resources in preventative measures and prenatal explorations of the emotional aspects of parenthood.

10
Journey to the Interior – Pre- and Perinatal Psychotherapy

'I may have had my baby by next session', says the woman on my couch, holding the rounded fullness of her belly. 'Next week I may be lying here with a new baby in my arms. What an amazing thought! ... But it won't really be new – the baby's been here all along, not just me . . . .'

The emotional demands of pregnancy and parenting are very great. In these last chapters we shall be looking at ways in which parents can benefit from psychoanalytic psychotherapy during pregnancy and the early months following the birth. Although it is written largely with psychotherapists or counsellors in mind, expectant couples or parents may also be interested to know more about such therapy.

I shall not be making a strict division between the pre- and postnatal periods, since an overlap often occurs. In the relatively new field of parent/infant therapy, I draw on work of pioneers and on my own cumulative experience of preconceptual, pre- and perinatal psychoanalysis and psychotherapy over the past two score years, in a clinical practice devoted to problems related to reproductivity. My work varies in frequency from one to five sessions a week, and ranges from relatively brief (6–18 sessions) to long-term (two to seven years) individual therapy and group work with many pregnant women.

People seek help themselves or are referred for a range of problems relating to general unhappiness, the pain of infertility, and/or the emotional impact of medical treatment; pseudocyesis ('imaginary' pregnancy); or conflicts during pregnancy, sometimes leading to abortion. Others present parenting problems such as bonding, feeding, sleep or separation difficulties, or abuse. An individual's distress may be directly related to childbearing – assisted conception; the demands of multiple babies; antenatal test results with negative implications; the anguish of miscarriage, stillbirth, prematurity, neonatal illness, or death. It may be triggered by major life events such as abandonment, separation, divorce; or bereavements during pregnancy or the early postnatal period; or a reaction to childhood deprivation; it may stem from exacerbation of chronic situations such as an unsatisfactory emotional or sexual relationship; economic hardships or life with an insensitive, alcoholic, or battering partner. Given the emotional upheaval around childbearing, any of these precipitators may trigger symptoms of varying degrees of severity and social impairment, such as anxiety, depression, perfectionism, eating disorders, substance abuse, delusional moods, anxiety or states of panic, feeling depersonalized during pregnancy or postnatally and dangerous to or persecuted by the fetus.

The majority of people in my caseload could be defined as neurotic or borderline, some with paranoid, schizoid, explosive, or obsessive-compulsive personality disorders. Because of the difficulty of containment in private practice and the risk to the infant, I have not accepted new referrals when frankly psychotic. In the few cases where psychotic features have emerged during the course of treatment, I have continued to see these patients, involving the GP, other members of the family, or back up provisions for the baby, as required.

Traumatic background factors contributing to current difficulties in some but by no means all people I have treated have included a childhood history of incestuous relationship(s), sexual, emotional and/or physical abuse; adoption, fostering or children's home placement as a child; being a 'replacement' child, illegitimate, deprived, orphaned or rejected. However, many people come from relatively intact and caring homes, although a high proportion have suffered previous unmourned abortion, miscarriage, or perinatal death in their own childbearing years or family of origin.

Melinda – a Clinical Example

Melinda, a childless woman aged thirty-two, started once-weekly therapy when she was eleven weeks pregnant. She was referred by her GP, whom her husband John (a policeman) had consulted because of her severe depression. He was worried because she had stopped going to her job as receptionist in an architectural office, and reported that he found her in bed during the day, although she was waking up very early.

Melinda complained she could not stop crying. She did not know why she was so unhappy, but she did feel hopeless and despairing about her ability to give birth. In the early sessions she was very tearful, and usually arrived late, looking dishevelled and feeling exhausted. She felt herself to be a terrible person totally unworthy of respect, and thinking I was watching her critically, often tried to censor her ideas to appease me. Nevertheless, she responded thoughtfully to interpretations, and her determination to procure a Caesarean lessened as she began to think about the pregnancy and became able to voice her fear of damaging the infant during labour, and her disbelief at being allowed to produce and keep a live baby.

With time, Melinda began to feel safer about exploring her 'nebulous' feelings, spent less of the session in tears, and began to voice a greater variety of emotions. She described her depression as a sense of 'caving in', which made her feel as if all the good things in life were lost forever. Gradually, it emerged that her inability to contemplate becoming a mother, let alone imagining the baby inside her, was related to deepseated guilt about an abortion she had had in her late teens. At the time, the abortion had seemed the only sensible solution to an impossible situation, but it had come back to haunt her 'with a vengeance' when, at twenty-eight, she found herself unable to conceive in her marriage.

Feeling he would reject her if he knew, Melinda did not tell John about her past, but the secret felt like a barrier between them. Blaming herself for their infertility, she was convinced she was being punished for her 'sin', and comforted herself with secret eating and vomiting binges, as she had throughout her life. These in turn increased her sense of failure, and anxiety that she was damaging her capacity to reproduce. Now, finally pregnant following years of fertility treatment, Linda felt unentitled to bear the baby whose sibling she had destroyed so 'casually'. She oscillated between eating compulsively in order to compensate the baby for her internal badness and to replenish her own depleted resources, and engaged in punitive purging and bulimic practices intended to negate her secret self-indulgence.

By now, Melinda had gone back to work part-time, and had increased her sessions to twice a week. Together, we worked through some of her distressing feelings; she had begun to feel the baby moving and was deeply worried about her capacity to sustain the pregnancy and nurture an infant.

Associations to a nightmare about a dead kitten inside a fridge brought back a forgotten memory from her third year, when Melinda's (Regulator) mother suffered a late miscarriage, and the regimented little girl unconsciously blamed herself for having caused it through her tantrums and desire to be the only child. Her mother said it was a boy, as she believed the aborted baby might have been. In fact, she now recalled that her depression had descended during her current pregnancy like a 'thick black cloud' after the ultrasound technician thought the baby was male. She feared her strong emotions would kill this 'kitten' too, or he'd kill her.

Melinda's depression altered to become a process of mourning the lost babies, when a further 'forgotten' fact emerged. Musing about her mother's total preoccupation with Melinda's younger brother, born within a year of the miscarriage, she realized that he was quite clearly a replacement baby, not only for the miscarried one but for the mother's own father who had died the previous year. In fact, Melinda's brother was named after him, and she recalled numerous incidents from her childhood when she had swallowed back her envy at his special position in the family because of her fear that he too would die like her ungrieved beloved grandfather. Gradually, a picture was drawn of an inhibitedly jealous and contrite little girl, always on her best behaviour, striving desperately to please and feeling abandoned by her 'cool' mother who overtly preferred her son, whom she breastfed 'constantly', to both daughter and husband.

As she grew older, recognizing their marital incompatibility, Melinda had felt the need to act as go-between for her increasingly estranged parents, alternating feeling sorry for each in turn and trying hard to bring about a reconciliation. She felt her father to be neglected by her detached mother, who saw him as tempestuous and critical of her. Melinda tried but felt unable to win his affections, although he was attentive when she was unhappy, and they shared a passion for cream cakes, in which they indulged secretly, as her austere mother disapproved. Increasingly, he spent long stretches away from home, and then revealed in a stormy outburst during her adolescence that he had been having a long-term, secret affair. Melinda now wept as she recognized how her teenage fling with a married man enacted her Oedipal desires, as well as being an abortive bid for freedom from the increasingly oppressive home atmosphere, and a search for the paternal, as well as maternal, love she craved.

Expiating her secret abortion, Melinda had become entrenched in serving as scapegoat for her now separated mother, while her brother won the glittering prizes and public praise. Becoming aware in her therapy of the interlacing dynamics in her family of origin that had kept her embroiled in her parents' lives rather than fully living her own, Melinda began experiencing her long-stifled rage and sadness at the wasted years. Examining her own marriage, she found her own needs interlocked unhealthily with those of her long-suffering, silently critical husband, who had grown up in a household with a depressed mother whom he had ineffectively protected from his violent stepfather. Although refusing to be referred for marital therapy or seek help in his own right, with the ripple-effect from Melinda's therapy their collusion lessened as she became more robust in herself and able to counter his doom-laden sense of imminent disaster with a new feeling of optimism. During the last weeks of her pregnancy both began to attend antenatal classes and, looking forward to the birth, the partners worked together to create a pretty nursery.

Following the birth of their son, which John attended, Melinda's therapy continued and new issues arose, relating to feeding difficulties and both parents' fears in dealing with the baby's crying and distress. Their respective anxieties and inability to trust little Aidan's capacity to survive the night without their intervention made it hard for them to put the baby down to sleep in his own bed without frequent checking on his breathing and over-rapid response to night waking. Melinda tended to feel persecuted but soothed the baby by feeding him at all hours of the night resentfully while John would dash to the crib and carry the baby around when he cried, jiggling him in what Melinda described as 'silent fury'. Exhaustion followed.

As Aidan grew more sociable his father started feeding him (solids). Although relieved, Melinda felt physically jilted, and intense sibling rivalry surfaced once again in Melinda in relation to Aidan's budding relationship with his father. In time she recognized how in the guise of being helpful she was in fact intervening to interrupt formation of a close contact between them. In the sessions we had concrete evidence of Melinda's ambivalent relationship to food, as I watched her subtle misinterpretation of three-month-old Aidan's signals as she expertly spoonfed him when he opened his mouth to protest, to the point of regurgitation.

Although the couple's capacity to communicate had improved, Melinda still found herself inexplicably jealous and low at times, and there remained unspoken tensions between the partners. Sexual incompatibilities lasted for months following the birth, as she felt unattractive when John ignored her sexually, but 'pulled in two' by the conflicting demands on her still-breastfeeding body when he wanted to make love. Linking this conflict to identification with her mother, and the conflicting loyalties she experienced as a child in relation to her parents, Melinda felt able to explore fears of her own burgeoning feelings more fully in therapy, and later in relation to her son/husband. Having continued to bring the baby to her weekly sessions until he was seven months old, she established a babysitting arrangement with another mother while she took a training course in draughtsmanship. At this time Melinda's sexuality came back into focus in the sessions, with emphasis on difficulties relating to sexual enjoyment and her overweight body. The work continued . . .

What I wish to illustrate in this example and below is how in the course of therapy, even on an infrequent once- or twice-weekly basis, new complexities unfold at different stages of the childbearing process, resonating with emotional issues in each of the partners. Resolution and integration may facilitate the emergence of other layers of difficulties, as well as newfound strengths to deal with these. Increasingly, as it is internalized, psychodynamic understanding may be seen to be applied to practical daily issues in the family between sessions, as well as enabling personal exploration of less-conscious intrapsychic pressures and interpersonal forces through live experience of feelings transferred into the consulting room.

Pregnancy and Psychoanalytic Psychotherapy

Despite its ubiquitousness, there has been relatively little written about treatment of pregnant women with psychoanalysis and psychoanalytic psychotherapy. A controversy exists as to whether psychodynamic treatment is beneficial, ineffective, or even detrimental during pregnancy. In my own clinical experience, for the majority of referrals therapy can be rich and rewarding, although treatment during the pregnancy differs somewhat from work with people referred at other times.

I use the terms 'pre-' and 'perinatal' psychotherapy to refer to work with individuals who come with problems specifically related to childbearing. It is useful to differentiate between patients who are already in treatment when they conceive, and those referred during pregnancy with infertility problems.

Women who become pregnant during the course of an ongoing analysis or psychotherapy experience an emotional shift due to inner turbulence and greater accessibility of unconscious material. This usually steps up the therapeutic process productively, the trajectory of which now becomes focused on this pregnancy and its meaning to this particular woman at this time. Inevitably, even for the patient who has achieved a fluidity of free association in her sessions, there may be specific resistances due to fantasies of the baby 'listening in'. Similarly, anxieties about its being affected both by her own disclosures and the analyst's verbalizations emerge and require interpretation. Competitiveness may become evident, with jealousy over the therapist's attentiveness to the emotional needs of the woman's baby self, and references to those of the baby she is carrying within her.

Expectant parents who actively seek psychoanalysis or psychoanalytic psychotherapy tend to do so with an air of urgency, due to reactivated vulnerabilities, panic aroused by the state of pregnancy itself, heightened anxiety and fears about the birth, or anticipated failing as a mother or father. These women and men are usually highly motivated although often ambivalent about therapy, which nevertheless can be extremely rewarding if primitive defences are overcome. Referrals often include people who would not usually seek or even know about psychotherapy, and those who have long denied a need for help.

In their pregnantly labile state, even brittle and manically defended women might touch a depth of emotion during the initial interview, which can be tested out with a probing interpretation, and if they prove insightful despite resistance, may be built upon in future meetings, going at their own pace. However, others take flight during the initial sessions or by repeated nonattendance indicate a lack of commitment to ongoing psychoanalytic psychotherapy at this time. Nevertheless, given the all-pervasive influence of a parent's unconscious over the baby, even a slight shift in a pathological stance may have long-lasting benefits, not least by provision of an alternative parenting model.

Supportive work might be indicated providing an authentic experience of having being listened to and understood. And when the door to therapy is kept open, people sometimes return at a time of greater readiness for change.

With satisfactory antenatal therapy, according to prior agreement work may end with some follow-up sessions after the birth. However, in the majority of cases during late pregnancy or following the birth a woman focuses feeling the need to be covered during the trials and tribulations of early motherhood, and asks for a new therapeutic contract to allow therapy to continue postnatally. In these cases flexibility of times and forebearance for unforseen changes, cancellations, and confusions are essential in the first six weeks, and some sessions might need to be curtailed to accommodate a fretful baby, or lengthened a few minutes until the end of a feed. Telephone exchanges might be necessary as a holding measure for postnatally depressed, agoraphobic, or highly anxious new mothers, and in desperate situations, some therapists practise home visits.

Assessment of Childbearing Patients

There are several peculiarities of assessment for therapy during pregnancy which may influence selection criteria otherwise applied. This is particularly true of expectant individuals/couples seeking therapy, who otherwise would have no inclination to do so.

Clinical assessment of pregnant women is at times affected by the florid presentation of primitive disequilibrium and primary process material, which may ring false alarms in the assessor. Conversely, facility of intuitive introspection may give a false reading of the woman's psychological-mindedness and long-term capacity to aggregate insight and integrate understanding. Similarly, narcissistic defences of grandiosity or idealization can be masked as a 'brilliant' pregnancy. Furthermore, the therapist's sense of ethical responsibility towards the unborn child might induce him or her to take on for psychoanalytic therapy an expectant parent who does not have the capacity to make use of psychoanalysis or psychoanalytic psychotherapy, but nevertheless could benefit from some other form of treatment such as supportive counselling, group work, or brief problem-focused psychotherapy, or cognitive treatment in the case of incapacitating phobias. It is therefore important for the psychoanalytical psychotherapist who is unable to vary her or his own technique to make a correct assessment and refer elsewhere people who would benefit more from other forms of treatment at this crucial time.

Nina Coltart, who arguably has conducted more diagnostic interviews for psychoanalytic treatment than most other psycho-analysts, draws attention to the crucial distinction between the 'will to be analyzed' and the 'wish for recovery'. She suggests the difficult discrimination between the two may surface in an initial interview by temporarily going against the patient's positive transferential feelings towards the interviewer with a confronta-tional interpretation. I find that this distinction between the need for understanding as opposed to symptom reduction may during pregnancy be expressed as a desire to become a better mother rather than a wish to 'feel better'.

In my view, two essential criteria of aptitude for dynamic treatment are: *a sense of agency* – the patient's awareness of having some degree of responsibility for their own emotional predicament – and *the capacity for self-reflection* outside the ses-sions. This may manifest as a commonsense, untutored under-standing of their own defensive strategies and a wish for change. Awaiting parenthood, many present with a 'now-or-never urgency' and high motivation to change before birth. While motivation is not sufficient to ensure successful treatment, alongside curiosity and a desire to make meaning it can serve as fuel to sustain formation of a therapeutic alliance.

Paradoxically, while in general people who habitually 'park' the source of the problem elsewhere are poor candidates for psychotherapy, childbearing people who blame their own par-ents for all their troubles may nevertheless be trying to resolve their difficulties and come to terms with their own transition from child to parenthood. Preoccupation with their own early parenting is indicative of anxieties about parenting their own children. Studies of intergenerational patterns of attachment have shown that expectant parents' description of their early history is predictive of the future relationship: bland or idealized accounts in mothers of insecurely attached avoidant children, and con-fused, lengthy accounts of early parenting typify mothers of resistant, ambivalently attached children, as opposed to the thoughtful accounts of parents of secure children (see Fonagy).

My clinical experience suggests that for therapeutic work,

positive indications in an expectant parent would be signs of potential capacity for care and concern for another; empathic awareness of other people's feelings; and recognition of and a desire to understand the emotional effect of one's own actions on close intimates. Absence of such concern may reflect a psychopathic personality; or a narcissistic lack of awareness of the needs of others; or a strong detachment defensively blocking out traumatic early experiences or schizoid fear of the ill-effects of one's own love (rather than hatred). Although the latter two are amenable to psychoanalytic treatment, the former are much less so. Likewise, people with severely obsessional personality structures may resort during pregnancy to circular ruminations and rigidification of defences, feeling too threatened by the unstructured nature of free-association to make use of therapy at a time of such great external uncertainty and internal turmoil. As a general principle, *therapy during pregnancy is counterindicated where it raises the level of anxiety in an already anxious person rather than reducing it.* Supportive counselling might be a better option in these cases or a holding therapy throughout pregnancy and the initial period postpartum, with a view to more extensive work following the emotional abatement after the first six weeks, or when the parent feels ready.

Unique Features of Psychoanalytic Psychotherapy During Pregnancy

Unlike most individual psychotherapeutic situations, during pregnancy the sanctity of the therapeutic twosome of psychoanalyst and analysand is invaded by a third – the fetus, ever-present, listening in. Often it is the pregnant woman who experiences the fetus as an intruder, eavesdropping on confidential material, demanding attention from her or the therapist, diverting her from listening to herself, and preventing her from speaking what is on her mind for fear of harming it. In its intrusiveness, the fetus might represent a recalcitrant, disowned aspect of herself, an envoy or spy sent by her partner, a competitor, rival sibling, or her own silent baby self clamouring to be heard.

For some therapists it is disconcerting to have this hidden client within the patient, to whom some of their interpretations are addressed. In addition to modifications due to concern about the pregnant woman's response, the analyst may also be unconsciously wary of fetal reaction.

For the woman herself, especially after she experiences internal activity, an intensified need to differentiate between the fetus and a representation of her baby self becomes apparent. Nevertheless, not unfancifully, the birth may continue to be regarded as a time of personal rebirth, with attendant urgency (to which the therapist unconsciously responds) about completing psychic gestation in time for the physical event.

The rapidly changing shape of the pregnant woman may be disconcerting to the therapist, particularly if the woman has been in therapy for some time before conception occurs. As the sessions pass, the physically growing belly marks off time, beginning to represent psychological growth – or its absence – as the increasing bulk concretely illustrates the accumulating weeks of therapy, and decreasing number of weeks to the birth. (The postnatal counterpart is seeing the baby fill out or fail to thrive.)

From the analyst's overarching viewpoint, whatever the time-span of treatment, from the moment of 'conception', as the patient is referred or first enters the consulting room, *like pregnancy therapy is intended to end*. However, during treatment, paradoxically an illusion is created and sustained for a while that the analytic situation can go on indefinitely until the process is completed. In therapy during pregnancy, this naïve trust is interfered with by awareness of a timebound competing process of physical gestation. The therapeutic process may be prematurely escalated, delayed, miscarried or abortively terminated, by a momentum of urgency to achieve psychic birth or complete a cycle before the physical birth overshadows the natural trajectory of ongoing treatment. In real terms, although therapy might and often does continue after the birth, what comes after the watershed event of birth often constitutes a new and different chapter.

In the safety of the consulting room, it is usual for intense emotions from the past to be reactivated and transferred from earlier significant figures on to the therapist. For the pregnant woman, however, identification with the fetus heightens an atmosphere of primitive transference to the therapist, experienced as a benign or malevolent enveloping, maternal womb carrying the patient to rebirth. According to the affective climate of the transference, the therapist may be experienced as a generous placenta, feeding nutrients, metabolizing material and transforming it for the patient's growth, while disposing of waste products and encouraging development. Or she or he may be perceived as a depriving, stingy or potentially abortive mother, resenting her presence or diverting good resources away so the patient suffers from 'placental' insufficiency. The psychological birth may be envisaged in positive terms as a healing rebirth, or negatively as a premature expulsion, or impending termination of treatment.

Focal preoccupation in the transference on issues relating to gestation, maternal nurturance, orality, fusion, expulsion and autonomy reticulate a complex web of fantasies linking images of her internal mother with those of the mother she wishes or fears to become, and the mothering she receives from her therapist. Confusion is compounded by an interplay of triple identifications between self, mother and fetus, and it is incumbent on the therapist to tease out the multiple levels before the birth.

A difficult task for the therapist is that of maintaining an even-handed approach: treading the tightrope between interpretation of defences on the one hand and, on the other, preservation of the modicum of idealization necessary for primary maternal pre-occupation; exploring anxieties while also acknowledging a possible reality behind her fears; and preparing the woman for the unlikely but real chance of a less-than-optimal outcome.

Sustaining an atmosphere of abstinence defined as the hallmark of psychoanalysis and psychoanalytic therapy becomes more complicated with a pregnant woman. Treatment of an expectant mother, like all therapy, aims to help the patient maximize their own resources. In this case, it means enabling the woman to leave the consulting room and face the outside reality on her own – the vicissitudes of her pregnancy, labour, birth, and the daily trials of mothering of her child.

For the therapist it may be increasingly difficult to preserve neutrality as he or she feels drawn to pamper the heavily pregnant woman or compelled to protect the unborn child from maternal abuse, or the patient from her own envious or destructive impulses. A pregnant woman's smoking or eating disorders take on a different impetus for the therapist and, postnatally, watching a baby being dangled by the arm or fed lying flat, she or he may be sorely tempted to temper an interpretation with an offering of practical guidance, or to comfort a persecuted mother with a maternal hug.

In psychoanalytic treatment, unlike counselling and brief psychotherapy, emotional regression occurs, which coupled with speaking aloud from deep within themselves, causes the person on the couch sometimes to forget about time, space, and the existence of the actual therapist, startling visibly if an interpretation breaks the spell.

During late pregnancy, as the woman withdraws deeper into herself and focuses inward, she may have begun to avoid socializing in her external life as social communication feels laboured, and it is an effort to make herself intelligible. Her sessions provide a rare relief as she feels permitted, indeed encouraged, to say anything that comes into her mind without censorship. Doubly released from social communication, she will care little about being understandable to her listener, and communications may at times alarmingly resemble babble or manic poesis, albeit playful, tearful, and at times cuttingly insightful.

If she neither dreads revelation of her wildest fantasies, murderous feelings, and deepest ambivalence, nor worries about appearing too needy, a pregnant woman may indulge herself by taking her feelings to extravagant lengths. Women who are depressed during pregnancy seem to benefit from the experience of being given 'permission' by the therapist to explore in the safety of the session the murky depths of their shameful secret feelings – having at times to overcome the inhibition of speaking 'in front of' the fetus – and time to work on them, before the baby's birth, rather than being jollied by shocked well-wishers outside. However, anxieties about the birth or the baby's abnormality are treated more cautiously by both therapist and patients, as the possibility of them materializing in reality cannot be ruled out.

Countertransference Issues During Pregnancy

In parallel with the patient's unconscious transference of feelings from the internal world onto the therapist, the latter experiences a countertransference of unconscious processes aroused in response to the patient's communications, and especially to the patient's unconscious transmissions. This silent 'dialogue', as Paula Heimann came to call the reciprocal interplay of unconscious forces, is thus the joint product of interaction between a particular analyst and a particular patient, and serves as a specific auxiliary source of emotional understanding during the sessions.

Countertransference perhaps resembles the often empathic experiences a receptive mother has with her baby: she may find herself on the receiving end of unconscious transmissions, which prime her responsiveness to knowing what the infant is experiencing. The mother's countertransference also involves the recreation of subjective emotional states resonating with her own infantile repertoire, and the involuntary triggering of physiological reactions, particularly with a girl baby. Depending on the accessibilty of her early self, the mother may attribute her arousal to intuitive awareness of the baby's subtle cues, her own heightened sensibilities due to empathic identification with the infant, or projective insertions by the baby.

What I am suggesting is that in the consulting room, as in the nursery, both definition and responsive evocation of countertransference are influenced by the *degree to which the human, subjective, and gender overlap between analyst and patient is recognized*, which in turn determines where the analyst places herself in relation to her patient.

A female analyst working with a female patient may experience a host of countertransferential feelings that arise out of their primary female experience and imagery, their meshing or clashing feminine identifications. For the therapist working with reproductive issues, countertransference is heightened by the primal nature of the infertile or pregnant woman's preoccupations. Childbearing confronts us with the most fundamental universal questions: what is the difference between the sexes? where do babies come from? how are they made? as we face the mysteries of conception, gestation, transformation and preservation.

In the countertransference during childbearing, as in the transference, the body is everpresent. With these clients, the therapist becomes a first-row witness to the drama, often allocated a voyeuristic position, party not only to intimate details of the couple's sex life, but also of their innards. Before conception there may be daily accounts of changes in the quantity and motility of his sperm; the quality, number and progress of her ripening follicles; or subtle changes in vaginal mucous viscosity or menstrual flow.

The consulting room is filled with a host of fantasy baby apparitions. After conception, descriptions of the shapeliness of fetal features visualized on ultrasound screens; nausea, aches, and pains and the various symptoms of pregnancy on the couch might suddenly give way to painful contractions and goriness of an approaching miscarriage or a retrospective blow-by-blow account of an excruciating birth. Simultaneously, the therapist is a helpless bystander, riding intense emotional fluctuations of monthly cycles of hope and despair until conception and the long months of agonizing uncertainty awaiting the birth. As guardian of the future, the therapist must uphold faith in the creative process while at times the patient enters a despairing Hell of abandoned hope.

Particularly powerful transferential implants may be projected by the pregnant patient, with inducements for the therapist to feel like and enact the patient's parental figures, or even to surpass them. These pressures may at times mesh into existing tendencies in the therapist, and may be difficult to disentangle from her own impetus to protect the vulnerable woman. As with psychotic patients, the pregnant woman's rush of primitive bodily preoccupations, archaic preverbal communications and intense primitive emotions have a powerful impact on the analyst, possibly arousing disturbing latent material or sympathetic bodily symptomatology.

The therapist's dual loyalties, and at times contradictory responsibilities towards both patient and baby, create an internal tension between speaking to the fetus, the child-in-the-patient, or the potential mother. Especially during a first pregnancy, the analyst's awareness of the momentous demands of the maternal task ahead and complex needs of the real baby to come, joins forces with her internal pressures towards mothering the pregnant patient, or her offspring, and a sense of being pregnant with, anxious about, and wishing to nurture the expanding client, who is about to be reborn as mother.

Countertransferential feelings are inevitably coloured by awareness of the physical risks that the patient faces through invasive procedures, daily discomfort in pregnancy, and imminent pain of childbirth. Possibility of miscarriage, Caesarean section, stillbirth, congenital abnormalities, or perinatal complications abound, and often these anxieties reside in the analyst, partially invested in her for safekeeping by the patient who cannot tolerate exploring them, and partially resulting from the analyst's own internal desire to protect the client while recognizing her inability to do so, and the realistic need to prepare the patient for unlikely events while avoiding unnecessary pessimism or alarm. As with all such issues, self-scrutiny reduces the danger of acting out in the countertransference.

Finally, despite Bion's challenge to the analyst to allow herself to be unfettered by 'memory or desire', we cannot but bring into the consulting room our sense of a general continuity of the patient, even if she is physically changing before our very eyes. The permeable emotionality of pregnancy and easy accessibility of preconscious material may throw an analyst's countertransferential feelings into disarray, as time and again she is caught by surprise by the acuity of the patient's intuitive observations. Equally disconcerting are unfamiliar facets of the patient or transference reaction which suddenly spring up full blown. A fascinating aspect of analyzing the same patient through more than one pregnancy is the recurrence of themes which subside between gestations.

'It is a very remarkable thing,' says Freud, 'that the Unconscious of one human being can react upon that of another, without passing through the Conscious.' (1915, p. 194) We might say that to-ing and fro-ing between transference and countertransference, the interwoven fabric of the session is shot through with unconscious communications between those 'aboriginal' populations of both patient and analyst, with the analyst not only receiving but at times undoubtedly transmitting his or her own images and messages. The analyst's most difficult task is simultaneously to remain open and receptively available, while also consciously attempting to monitor and formulate these feelings.

In conclusion, distinctions may be drawn between countertransference reactions in a variety of different categories of therapists.

The childless psychoanalyst or therapist inevitably experiences disturbing twinges of envy and awesome appreciation of the powerhouse of live creativity on their couch. The sense of being in the presence of a mysterious, eternal and inexorable process may affect the humbled therapist's conviction of his or her own creative healing skills, a demotion which in turn interlaces with a sense of Oedipal triumph in the pregnant patient. Retriggered unconscious wishes for a child may be troubling or evoke a redoubled sense of failure in therapists who have themselves been subfertile.

For a parent-therapist, the focus on fecundity may arouse a sense of broodiness coupled with envy or relief at having moved beyond this phase. With a pregnant client, access to primitive emotions may re-evoke repressed or unresolved elements from a female therapist's own previous pregnancies, arousing her empathy, protectiveness, defensiveness, confusion or aversion, or complex envy in an adoptive parent, or male therapist.

For a pregnant therapist, with all her patients the swelling reality of her pregnancy interferes with neutrality by bringing her fertility and sexuality into the foreground of the therapeutic situations. This may be particularly poignant in relation to childless or infertile patients and those currently awaiting conception (although for some, the therapist's pregnancy is deemed to have contagious magical properties). As Ruth Lax demonstrated, each patient reacts differently to the therapist's pregnancy in accordance with reactivation of their own most significant infantile conflict. Issues of sexual curiosity, unconscious awareness of conception, sibling rivalry, jealousy of the fetus, envy of the therapist's fecundity, and competitive strivings with her virile partner have all been noted by various psychoanalysts and therapists such as Cecille Bassen, Sheri Fenster, Sue Gottlieb, Carol Nadelson and Linda Penn, and more recently Alicia Etchegoyen and Paola Mariotti, psychoanalysts who have candidly discussed their countertransferential feelings during their own pregnancies.

Little discussed is a double pregnancy: faced with a pregnant client and her fetus, the pregnant analyst introduces a fourth into the consulting room – her own fetus. Although she might wish to protect her baby from both work stresses and the raw emotions expressed in the session, she can only do so by reducing her own sensibilities. The pregnant therapist's vulnerability is increased while her concentration may be decreased. Self-absorption is disturbed by the rigorous demands of her work and conversely, attention is frequently diverted by nausea, tiredness, internal movements, contractions and fragments of fantasy. Listening to a pregnant patient she may be hard pressed by her own desire similarly to indulge in introspection as well as experiencing a need to maintain her own private experiences from being preempted or intruded upon. She may be loath to entertain a patient's uncertainty or anxieties about the baby's normality, or birth-fears which may trigger her own, tempting her to foster complacent optimism in self-protection. The analyst might indeed feel robbed of original reactions to her own pregnancy, or collude with the pregnant patient's competitiveness.

Clearly, her heightened emotionality can serve as a refined countertransferential tool. However, differentiation must be achieved between the therapist's subjective arousal due to her own pregnant upheaval and that of the client, a difficult task when both seismographs are quivering in unison.

In sum, pregnancy powerfully reactivates an arena of primitive emotions, resonating with each person's particular psychohistory – relating to the original reproductive parents, to passions of the primal scene, forbidden sexual knowledge and generative enigmas as well as high emotional tension between life-producing and death-dealing forces, fertile power and vulnerability. These potent themes come alive if either therapist or patient expect a baby. When both do, and pregnant therapist and pregnant patient come together in the rich climate of a single consulting room, transference-countertransference permutations are manifold.

Why Psychotherapy During Pregnancy?

The common thread running throughout this book is a variegated one composed of intertwisted strands of love and hate. Ambivalence is the stuff of connections, and the umbilical cord is no exception. As we have seen, pregnancy and early parenthood are times of heightened emotional lability and deep-seated sensitivity to internal and external excitations. To successfully negotiate the journey between being someone's child to becoming someone's parent, the pregnant woman and her partner, if she has one, will have to come to terms with mixed emotions and great shifts in the structuring of their sexual, couple, and personal identities. Although many expectant parents make the transition on their own, some need help to gain access to, recognize, and work through a past traumatic legacy and its reactivation in their present interactions. Therapy during pregnancy is a timely and cost-effective method of treating disturbances within one person before they become established conditions between two or more.

Economical considerations may also apply to the effectiveness of prenatal therapy in reducing the likelihood of postnatal depression and suicidal attempts, possibly preventing obstetric complications, and pre-empting the long-term effects of pathological parent-baby interaction, child abuse, and emotional neglect.

Throughout this book and elsewhere I have presented my observations on the many ways in which pregnancy urges re-evaluation of the expectant parent's integrity and internal world configurations, affecting psychological functioning and ideation, including increased permeability to magical thinking and primitive fantasies.

The widespread emotional disequilibrium of pregnancy has long been recognized in the psychoanalytic literature by old-timers such as Helene Deutsch, Thérèse Benedek, Grete Bibring, and, more recently, Judith Kestenberg and Dinora Pines. In addition, researchers have also noted proliferation of transient psychological symptoms reported in various studies, notably anxiety, depression, mood lability, and insomnia.

Pregnancy can thus be seen to act as a provoking factor for mental illness in women who are particularly vulnerable due to various risk factors, such as economic problems, marital difficulties, unplanned pregnancy, poor social support, and past psychiatric history. Bearing in mind the high prevalence of emotional disturbance and the common upsurge of primitive fantasies during pregnancy, and given ubiquitous attendance at antenatal clinics, in my view it is commonsense to offer therapeutic help, which should be made available particularly for vulnerable women at the time when they most need it. Ideally, health care professionals should be trained in rudimentary screening; antenatal clinics should offer discussion groups, and a counsellor or therapist should be made available to any woman who wishes to see one pre- or postnatally.

From a sociological point of view, Western women may be more at risk than their counterparts in traditional societies. As noted earlier, during pregnancy there is little recognition of the emotional upheavals and birth fears or fantasies, which are ritually catered to and ceremonially dispelled in other places. In stratified societies such as our own, new parents have rarely seen, let alone touched, a newborn before being given full and unsupervised responsibility for caring for the baby in isolation, without adequate training. It is common for antenatal parent-craft classes to focus on the practicalities of nappy-changing, bathing, and breastfeeding a doll, although these are rapidly learned with the live baby in hospital after the birth. However, the incredible emotional transition demanded of new parents and their vulnerability to postnatal depression are rarely, if ever, touched upon. Controlled trials of group therapy for expectant couples or pregnant women show improved relationships between the partners, reduction in birth complications, and less idealization postnatally (see Niemela). Similarly, studies evaluating transition-to-parenthood groups which emphasize emotional and social support have found a reduction in postnatal depression (see Leverton & Elliott, and Cowans).

Clinical observations of individuals having psychotherapy during pregnancy clearly demonstrate increased tolerance of their own anxiety and ambivalence after the birth, and greater awareness of emotional resourcefulness in dealing with the baby. In my own experience, I have found not only that pregnant women are suitable subjects for psychoanalysis or individual psychoanalytic psychotherapy, but many benefit from group therapy. From a psychosocial standpoint, apart from offering a pregnant woman an opportunity to work through her unconscious preoccupations, *group psychotherapy* with a variety of women during pregnancy provides a first-time mother with an emotional preview of motherhood, and familiarizes her with real newborns and their psychological needs, as women return to the group with their infants following the birth. Postnatally, the group often serves as an ongoing support group for mothers and babies during their most vulnerable time together.

The incidence of puerperal psychosis is similar worldwide at one in 500 to 1,000 births. In the West, however, there is a fivefold risk of neurotic illness in parents during the first year postnatally than in all the rest of our lives, and high percentages of mothers are found to be affected by postnatal depression, with up to sixty per cent experiencing mild depressive syndromes, and some six to twenty-eight per cent suffering severe depression. These figures vary crossculturally, seemingly with a much lower incidence in traditional societies. In industrialized Japan, which has managed to retain many time-honoured traditions alongside ultramodernization, the very low incidence of 'baby blues', but also of postnatal depression, has been attributed to the still prevalent custom of the new mother spending the first weeks following the birth in her mother's home.

Unaccountably, we have rarely taken prophylactic measures nor exploited preventive opportunities but wait to treat established conditions. I feel strongly that the widecast net of antenatal services should provide unusual opportunities for group work, befriending, identification and mental health screening of high-risk women, and referral for psychotherapeutic treatment, while well-baby clinics offer possibilities for postnatal follow-up and support groups. In some Scandinavian countries, linked to substantial incentives by way of maternity benefits, antenatal attendance at maternal health care centres, and postnatally at family health care centres has risen to almost one hundred per cent, and staff usually includes a psychologist. In the UK, health visitor services means that every family has personal care in the home from a professional. Recently it has been shown that, if trained to detect psychological problems, health visitors can be effective in reducing distress and promoting referral for treatment (see Holden). Similarly, in the last few years midwifery training has begun to include courses leading to greater understanding and recognition of psychological problems which manifest prenatally. (Studies, such as McNeil's, which have retrospectively relied on midwife interviews illustrate their intuitive capacity to note and appraise psychopathology quite accurately.) Clearly, both antenatal and perinatal primary carers should be trained to identify disturbance and make referrals for treatment. Antenatal therapeutic facilities are economically expedient and should be a high priority for individuals, couples, and high-risk parents and babies. Discussion groups for exploring the emotional concerns of pregnant women could be run simultaneously with antenatal checkups, and made available to all women attending clinics, staffed by a single psychologist, therapist, or a specially trained counsellor.

Traditional cultures provide a continuity of childbearing-lore and caregiving which has been eroded in our society. Professionals have stepped into the gap, although scarcity of trained personnel and economy cuts in provisions have reduced even those scant services which were previously available. In industrialized societies, given the amount of time spent by caregivers in relative isolation with their babies in nuclear families, it is imperative that health promoting resources are strengthened within the family itself.

To reiterate the advantages of psychotherapy during pregnancy as I see them:

- Emotional crises during pregnancy and motivation to become good parents propel people to seek help, including some who may otherwise have no wish for or interest in therapy.
- The urgency to complete treatment before the birth acts as a further inducement to overcoming resistances; many contracts are extended postnatally.
- Therapy can reduce the likelihood of obstetric complications, postnatal depression and child abuse by providing time and space to explore distress and unconscious anxieties in preparation for the baby, parenthood and the birth.

- Psychotherapy during pregnancy can serve as a healing experience for deficits in an expectant parent's own childhood, offering an opportunity to break transgenerational patterns by working through unconscious conflicts and revitalized issues, rather than enacting them with the next generation.

PRE- AND PERINATAL TREATMENT GUIDELINES

	Nature of Disturbance RECOMMENDED TREATMENT		
	Crisis	**Transition**	**Chronic**
	CRISIS INTERVENTION/ DEVELOPMENTAL GUIDANCE	BRIEF DYNAMIC THERAPY	PSYCHOANALYTIC PSYCHOTHERAPY
INFANT	fetal abnormality failure to thrive	reactive disorders	handicap deprivation
	sessions*: 1-3	3-5	5+
FAMILY INTERACTION	sexual impasse sleep disturbances feeding problems	bereavement prematurity immigration	dysfunctional family emotional discordance neg. representations
	sessions*: 2-4	4-8	8+
MOTHER	abortion conflict anxiety re: labour/birth work decisions	miscarriage panic reactions reactive depression	anxiety low self-esteem anorexia substance abuse persecutory thoughts
	sessions*: 3-6	6-10	25+

FOCUS OF THERAPY

*Approximate duration of therapy

11
Therapy in Early Parenthood

As it is my patients from whom I have learned most of what I know, it is apt that I begin the concluding chapter with the words of one whom we have met several times before:

> 'I was thinking about the baby in the womb needing something to push against . . .', she says after a silence, lying on the couch holding her pregnant belly. 'With my mother there's nothing there. If I push I get nothing in return, either she caves in or goes beserk . . . nothing firm to push against that recognizes my individuality, or counters in an elastic, resilient way – it's like hitting a punctured balloon. It's left me with no strong sense of myself impinging on others, as if she has no internal homespun trust in either herself or me. She just collapses or cites an external authority who 'knows' what's done.
>
> 'Daniel's a delight these days. We have short-lived trantrums when he's tired or hungry or jealous of the baby, but usually no run-ins. Am I too lax? I don't know. We sort it out between us, or he goes off to his room until he cools off. Most of the time when we play he's being a Tyrannosaurus, and such fun to be with! Trouble is, I get very tired, whereas he has masses of energy and curiosity, and if I let him do everything with me – cook and clean and all – he'd be on top of the world. But my main failing is that sometimes I have to put on a video for him when I need to do something myself quickly . . .
>
> 'It's surprising to see how clear it is that *what has been good for me here in analysis is good for him too*; not two different laws, but enough time to develop at my own pace, and being treated as an individual . . . being trusted and given respect and acknowledgement, being listened to and understood, and finding for one's self what feels right. It all applies to him. I can hear my mother's voice saying, "That path leads to a spoilt, bohemian child – one of those creative, renegade, obnoxious kids". But my main fear is of him becoming as regulated as I was. I'd rather he was cheeky than compliant and down-trodden or miserable . . . I suppose it's a question of trusting him to find his own path and going along with him,

rather than pulling him along a predictable path to become the person he *has* to be.'

Becoming a parent energizes connections between the generations, heightening awareness of emotional correspondence and differences in a mother or father's relationship to her or his own parents, dead or alive. Exposure to the arousing rawness of the newborn's emotions throws up a host of disturbing unconscious experiences for reappraisal, as well as the new and demanding adjustments of parenting.

Therapy in early parenthood differs according to the location of the problem – whether centred within the person referred, or necessitating joint therapy. Individual therapy during early parenting gives the caregiver time and a safe space for reflection away from the fray, enabling him or her to think not only about the ongoing interaction with the infant and partner, but within the internal world from a perspective of self-observation. We may say that the therapist creates a *hierarchy of holding* in which the securely held parent is able to experience, identify, and process his or her own infantile feelings and in turn can empathically help the infant to deal with overwhelming emotions. Clarification of their anxieties often changes not only parental feelings and behaviour in relation to the baby's feeding patterns or sleep and separation problems, but filters through to other members of the family.

However, sometimes the therapist finds she is only dealing with one part of the equation, and the partner in difficulty – whether the baby, another child, or caregiver – is conflating disturbance and resisting or blocking healthy change. In such cases, referral of the adult partners for a specialist consultation may lead to couple therapy or individual therapy of the other partner, or to child therapy for a sibling. Alternatively, it may be necessary to instigate parent/infant therapy centred on that pair's interchange, or for the whole family to be seen for brief therapy, focusing on disturbances in their interaction as a unit.

As illustrated throughout this book babies have a powerful influence over care givers. In some parents they arouse tenderness, and sometimes feelings of desperation. When these revitalized early emotions are too traumatic or uncontained, they create internal reverberations which affect the adult's parenting capacities. Conversely, we have become more aware of the extraordinarily powerful capacity of care givers to unconsciously recreate the baby of their own internal preconceptions. This happens not by magical means, but through emotional reinforcement of certain aspects of exchange with the baby and non-responsiveness or punitive reactions to others, resulting in extinction or suppression of that which they wish to avoid. When the parent's inside story spills out over the infant, he or she is made to play a part in its enactment. Perverse or highly restricted representations of the baby manifest in pathological interactions leading to disturbances in the development in the infant's self-image (of which the parent may be oblivious).

Intergenerational transmission of problems may be halted by psychotherapeutic treatments for parents who become aware of needing help or are referred when they are incapacitated by depression, agitation, rigidity, or hypochondriachal anxiety, or else referral is made because someone has become alarmed by the baby. By providing a safety valve, therapy eases the current situation, aiming to enable the patient to formulate their own painful and sometimes repressed traumatic childhood experiences and deprivations in words rather than somatic or behavioural enactments. Sometimes, when the parent is temporarily inaccessible to interpretation, careful use of video-feedback or verbal commentary on play or physical handling of the infant in the presence of the therapist can mitigate phobic feelings.

Such de-sensitization can be crucial if the parent is incapacitated by fear of their own or the baby's bodily excretions and explosive feelings, and also helps to de-eroticize touch and intimacy. In cases of failure to thrive, neglect, or abuse, crisis intervention may be necessary. In some mother/infant therapies such as pioneered by Selma Fraiberg and her team, brief treatment takes place in the child's home with developmental guidance accompanying therapy during critical situations. This may supplement intensive treatment in infant mental health clinics with at-risk babies. Such treatments, and those of mother/infant psychoanalytic psychotherapists, aim to alleviate chronic relational and/or behavioural disturbances due to the baby's mental or physical handicaps or pathological environments. Positive exchange between parent and baby gradually increase as the mother and/or father discover the baby to be rewarding rather than persecuting and become more aware of discrepancies between the real infant and their own negative internal representations.

Some therapists focus on areas of specific difficulty (crying, feeding, sleep, contact, communication); others take a more generalized approach to the interaction. In my own work I do not structure the situation in any way, but when relevant I elicit comments on an exchange between mother and baby as I might about a dream, or interpret the mother's actions in the light of my familiarity with aspects of her internal world. In a small minority of cases, particularly with depressed or estranged mothers, I may film a few moments of their exchange and replay the video to illustrate the degree to which she may be missing the baby's cues and signals:

'My baby never looks at me', complains a depressed mother. Watching the brief fragment of video she becomes aware of the frequent subtle mismatch of their rhythms as she consistently turns to her baby *after* he has tried to engage. The video shows how recurrently he focuses on her, concentrating with increasing puzzlement, then, frowningly, averts his gaze and limply gives up hope of reciprocity, which is the point at which she glances at him and finds him unresponsive.

Similarly, unconscious bipolar conflicts in a mother's orientation can be illustrated to the mother:

Jane, in once-weekly therapy, has been very permissive in breastfeeding her baby. However, the notion of weaning connects with her fragile self-esteem. As solids are introduced, she is unaware of her ambivalence, but begins to regulate her child's eating, and the video picks up the way she misreads signs of ongoing eagerness, interrupting his feed to unnecessarily wipe the baby's chin throughout the meal, spooning too fast, and commiserating when he chokes, and showing him his food then abruptly closing the jar midway despite his protest. Seeing herself enables Jane to contemplate how rejected she feels when he seems to prefer processed food to her own milk.

In subsequent sessions, Jane becomes aware of her anxiety of my dismissing her if she becomes independent, and can think more about her fears of being thrust aside as her baby grabs at a rich and varied diet of interaction which she feels unable to provide. She fears not being valued for her intrinsic worth, and her lifelong sense of having to curtail her own desires to validate her facilitating mother's excellence. As her baby approaches his first birthday, Jane, aware of external pressure to wean him, succumbs to internal conflicts and once again becomes increasingly inconsistent, severely forbidding snacking between meals, encouraging yet interfering with self-feeding, abruptly dropping breastfeeding at bedtime, but relenting at midnight and even waking him to feed.

Observations of mother-baby couples conducted by every psychoanalytic psychotherapy student in the course of their training, and neonatal research have greatly increased our understanding of the complex interpersonal matrix in which the baby acquires a sense of self.

In a handful of cases over the years, where this has proved non-disruptive to the therapy, for research purposes I have introduced regular video-taping for a short period of each session, from birth onwards. One copy of the complete tape is given to the mother as a record of the baby's development, the other is used for analysis of the couple's interactions. Having access to the mother's internal world through ongoing therapy, her need to make emotional sense of her experience and unprompted expression of heart-felt exchanges during sessions gives these recordings a different weighting to those made under ordinary baby observation conditions or in laboratories. In them, continuity of the habitual interactional climate of a particular mother-baby from birth is apparent (and in some cases may be compared to the same mother with another of her babies). Similarly, the infant's fine-tuned capacity for matching moods and sharing maternal affective states become evident, as well as temporary discrepancies in mutual receptivity, when one partner is engrossed in salient emotions. For example, here is a two-minute segment taken in my consulting room:

> Kevin, aged fourteen weeks, is sitting in his chair facing his mother, who sits crosslegged on the carpet, shading him from the sunshine streaming in at the window. Both are colourfully dressed; he is wearing little red socks, and throughout the mother absentmindedly cups his feet and passes them from hand to hand as she speaks to me. He turns from watching the

flashing red light on the video camera near me back to his mother, with an open mouthed crow 'A-eio'. She interrupts what she's saying to me, about having just appointed a nanny, to pitch her voice higher, as she smilingly says to me through him, 'Wonderful sounds . . . he giggles and chats . . .'. She says this cooingly, then continues to me in a deeper voice, 'I was in the lounge feeling terribly bereft. [There was] nothing to stop me going in, but I wanted her to establish a relationship, but then a feeling . . . of not sharing that moment . . .' 'Envy of their contact?', I suggest. Kevin turns at the sound of my voice, smiles at me, then turns back to beam at his mother, but then, flashing her a quick look, begins to watch her rather warily, seemingly aware that her expression has changed.

'It was a sense more of loss rather than jealousy. I was losing out . . . This morning feeding him [he was] much more interested in [the] concept of my preparing food than eating it . . .' She has speeded up, seemingly in response to his concern, and adds in a higher-pitched aside to Kevin, accompanied by a little laugh, 'Very excited about mashing banana and *mango*'.

She raises her intonation; Kevin squeaks with delight, smiling, looking at me, then intently back at his mother, as if waiting for more. Her voice drops again. '[I] spend very little time feeding him. . . Up at five-thirty, breakfast after two hours . . .' Kevin says a high-pitched 'Aah', watching his mother closely, face raised towards hers. She bends forwards; he repeats 'Aahh', slightly more prolonged this time; she says animatedly: 'I know! I *know*! . . . Had a good sleep?', then something inaudible, and she lowers her tone and slows her voice again to continue talking to me, still holding his gaze and his foot. '. . . and thinking how *silly* it is to miss out on all that . . . I went in to work on Tuesday for an hour and left her [the nanny]. [He] got a bit fractious in the afternoon, and I could hear him with her learning what makes him settled, and I kept thinking [Kevin turns to me] I *know* how to settle him.' Kevin's gaze goes back to mother, past her, to the window beyond. 'Which isn't entirely true, but going *away* – the separation's horrible. When I'm away from him, I'm all right.' Kevin's look bypasses her again, sweeping across her to watch me or the video light intently. '. . . *think of him* and coming home and I did resist ringing home for a couple of hours' [joke in her voice], 'and then the new anxiety I've never had before of getting home to him in time to give him his feed and his bath.' Kevin, who has drooped a little revives at her joke. Saying 'Mmm' he stretches, still facing me, and raises his right arm curved above his head. Mother pauses, then continues, her voice now plaintive. '. . . and he just seems . . . everyone says, "Oh, you'll get used to it", I'm sure I will, but it seems *so* sad.' Kevin gazes quickly at mother, then yawns full-mouth, eyes straight ahead. He looks directly at her eyes; she laughs a little forlornly; he turns to face in my direction; pauses, stretches with a half-yawn towards her, checks her face, saying 'Mmmm.' She replies 'Mm'; tries smiling tearfully. '. . . and I hate him to see me crying.' She sighs; he faces me briefly with another yawn and stretch, then keeps his gaze intently on her as she sniffs. 'It just seems rather silly to go through all that anxiety to have him . . . [her voice frankly tearful] . . . 'I know. I *know* I wouldn't be much good home all day long [inaudible] . . . things to do.' Scratches her crotch, putting both his feet momentarily in one hand to do so. 'But equally, so sad to leave him for *such a long time* . . . I felt that all the way through the pregnancy and breastfeeding . . .'

In addition to illustrating the infant's fine-tuned responsiveness to subtle changes in the mother's emotional state, this fragment also clearly demonstrates the dilemma of having a baby present in a therapy session. However, for a woman who is reluctant to leave her baby, at times that seems the only option.

Postnatal Treatment

Life with a new baby is a constant, often exhausting round of activities, and many new parents have little space to talk about their own hectic emotions. Pregnancy, labour, and birth require psychic digestion and integration, at the very time when the arrival of a new member of the family, who has to be assimilated, has a further emotional impact on the external and internal worlds of the parent. These tasks cannot be accomplished without the thoughtful capacity to engage.

Apart from patients who begin therapy from, during, or before pregnancy, some people refer themselves or are referred soon after the birth of a baby with problems they clearly relate to the ricochet effect of exposure to primitive emotions. Their difficulties may take the form of postnatal depression, or feature as persecutory anxieties; intrusive, violent, or sexual thoughts; or impulsive actions, detachment, and inability to relate to the baby. In some cases, these may be presented as specific management problems ('My baby never sleeps a wink!'), but reflect parental feelings around wider issues of separateness and separating (see, for instance, Dilys Daws). Brief psychotherapy may centre on crying, feeding, maternal guilt over employment, inability to establish satisfactory sleep patterns, or painful practical diffi- culties faced by bereaved parents or those with premature, chronically ill, or retarded babies.

However, all these problems, and the need to come to terms with a difficult birth or breastfeeding failure, must be seen in the context of the parents' psychic reality, wider relationships, and past emotional history.

Intimate relationships are regularly found to deteriorate fol- lowing the birth of a new baby. Couples or individuals often arrive in therapy to resolve a crisis in their emotional relation- ship, in which sexual disturbances and realignment of resources usually feature. Unlike psychotherapeutic treatments ongoing from pregnancy, or those that began even before conception, with referrals during the early postnatal period treatment must focus is primarily on urgent interpersonal difficulties and current disturbance between parents and/or baby, while exploring the contributing factors in the parents' own internal stories.

In individual or couple therapy, as each person comes to own their own past and present emotional experiences, and 'takes back' their projected bits, the burden is lessened for the baby or partner who has been used to siphon it off or express it indi- rectly. In some couples, partners may have become unable to co-operate supportively, as turmoil has been dealt with by seg- regating gendered functions and caregiving into good and bad figures: 'He hasn't got a clue what to do with the baby. He's just like my horrible father was – all butterfingers and rudeness. I don't let him anywhere near the child.' Joint therapy may lessen rigid ascriptions. When presented as a specific problem, such as colic or disturbed sleep, seemingly located in the baby, exploration of parental inability to set limits, to tolerate the baby's distress, or to believe in the infant's capacity to survive or function without the parents' total devotion day and night, may reveal internal configurations underpinning behaviour (extreme Facilitator/Participator). Other difficulties stem from parents defending against the fear of being sucked in to the whirlpool of reactivated infantile emotions through detachment, regimentation, and avoidance of empathy with the infant, or a rigid inability to recognize and respond to his/her emotional signals (extreme Regulator/Renouncer).

Reduction of unconscious stereotyping, and acknowledging their right to a sexual relationship which neither seduces the child nor allows him or her to keep them apart, can also strengthen the partners in their parental alliance. By using therapy to come to know their own strengths, weaknesses, and internal resources, self-assurance is increased as is the parents' capacity to trust the baby's resources and accept emotions without fear of uncontrollable escalation.

With expectant or new parents in therapy one generally finds a paradoxical situation: while fostering a process of emotional change that may involve regression before they can take responsibility for thinking about the causes of disturbance, the therapist must aim to activate their healthy adult resources, bearing in mind that the parents continue to have full charge of the baby between sessions. Simultaneously, the security of therapy can enable the parent to catch up on what they feel they have missed in the course of their own infancy, in the service of parenting, thus coming to provide for their own baby without envy. Finally, as in all psychoanalytic therapy, revival in the transference of emotional experiences with parental and other significant figures provides a live arena for reworking the past, rather than replaying it passively or actively within the new family setting.

The Presence of the Baby in Therapy

Psychotherapeutic treatment may involve mother and father jointly, or else one or both may be seen separately, with or without the baby. The presence or absence of the baby in the sessions is partly determined by the nature of the problem, parental decision, and practical arrangements. No doubt there are psychoanalysts or therapists who categorically declare the baby an obstruction in therapy; others may feel strongly that the baby should not be left by the mother during the first months, and therefore either therapy must be postponed or the baby brought along.

To my mind, whether the baby comes to therapy or not is a question that must be examined by each mother and therapist at various points in time, and must take account of both internal and external realities. Bringing the baby may serve a healthy function of the mother sharing her pride or her sorrows: showing the therapist her 'produce'; asking for help with difficulties; feeling gratified by the 'grandparental' admiration; seeking experience of a rejected baby or aspect of her own baby self; and permission to nurture. For some people, therapy provides the only experience they have ever had of honest, uninhibited, self-expression, bringing everything to one place and having both good and bad feelings genuinely recognized, simultaneously.

In couple therapy, the safe consulting room and presence of a strong third person may provide an opportunity to speak openly of issues that remain suppressed at home. Observing the partners' interaction at close range provides the therapist with useful information about the quality of contact between the couple, and of each towards the baby. If tolerated, outbursts and intense moments of emotional interchange can be fruitfully interpreted, and transformed into a catalyst for change. However, with malfunctioning parents who are less accessible to interpretation, video replays demonstrate use of body language, disturbed or effective sequences of interaction between themselves or with the baby, without breaking the flow. Skilful therapists can provide that mirroring function by intervening verbally and taking the couple back through their paces to show how the baby is being miscast or exploited to enact unexpressed aspects of the adult(s).

Sometimes the baby's presence may be used by parents as a defensive screen. They may interact with or through the infant to avoid relating to each other or making direct contact with the therapist. Others tacitly encourage the baby or toddler to create a situation which prevents any meaningful verbal exchange taking place. In some cases, the baby's presence acts as a barrier to parental disclosures of their own suffering or ambivalence for fear of affecting the child. As we observed earlier in the session with Alice's mother and Kevin's here, even very young babies are acutely aware and troubled by maternal distress or heightened emotionality. In situations where the baby acts as a parental inhibitor or is at risk of being disturbed by the proceedings, the therapist must insist on seeing the adult patient alone at least some of the time.

Conversely, women who have been having therapy or analysis during or before pregnancy often go to great lengths to exclude the baby from the sessions, feeling that their own baby self will affect the baby, or, conversely, be intruded upon by the real infant's presence: 'This is *my* time, my special time for myself. No sharing!' For many women the time spent with the psychotherapist may be their only time away from the baby; as such it constitutes space for reflection, and a means of gaining perspective outside a home situation which may be perceived as gruelling. When problems relate to interaction with the baby, however, therapy is enhanced by the presence of the child; or when the mother is reluctant to separate, or has no facilities to leave her baby elsewhere, it is the therapist's responsibility to make suitable provisions – of safety, comfort, warmth, toys, and changing facilities, or access to crèche or temporary minder – which must vary to keep pace with the growing child's needs.

What and where?

Postnatal therapy is in its infancy, born of increasing awareness of the importance of the early mother-baby exchange. Following the pioneering efforts of psychoanalysts such as Anna Freud, Donald Winnicott, Melanie Klein, and John Bowlby, support and help for parents, and therapeutic provisions for children, have gradually become more prevalent.

Whenever help is offered, and whatever it consists of, new parents need to find a safe context in which they can have the space and wider perspective to make sense of their distressing experience, which at times threatens to overwhelm them with inexplicable emotions. As we have seen throughout this book, close-range, unremitting exposure to an infant for whom one has life-and-death responsibility evokes echoes of an inside story, powerful narratives and primitive, inchoate memories from a time when the parent him- or herself was a helpless child at the mercy of a seemingly omnipotent mother or father. When these feelings are left unexplored, emotional and sexual abuse, neglect and violence may be perpetuated, as each successive generation is drawn unerringly unconsciously to project, repeat, and physically enact crucial emotional climates and the relationships from their internal realities, actualizing and inflicting these on those closest to them.

Models of Parenting and Therapy –
The Interactional Climate

In the view I have put forward in this book, psychological formation takes place not in isolation but within a two- or three-person interpersonal situation. I have suggested that our subjective internal worlds, cognitive abilities, and personalities begin to crystallize in the context of understanding others and being understood and recognized. This takes place with care givers who respond with the full sum of their subjective experiences and unconscious configurations – the combined, distinctive features of which constitute what I have termed the interactional 'climate' of the early exchange. It is aspects of this climate that become reactivated in the therapeutic transference, and in close relationships.

My colleague Christopher Bollas coined the evocative phrase the 'unthought known' to describe the unprocessed knowledge which we unconsciously possess but have never articulated into consciousness. Putting words to these unconsciously known, but unthought-out thoughts in therapy is a function of mental processing. I have found that for some people, the breakthrough flooding of unconscious, unprocessed, and unintegrated mental states that occurs during pregnancy and early parenting requires a metabolizing care giver to complete the unfinished process.

Therapy provides a reflective space for parents to step out of the emotional turmoil of their parenting situation and reflect on the powerful, nebulous feelings aroused in them by exposure to the primitive emotions in their infant. In this way the therapist enables the mother or father to give shape and meaning to their own infantile emotions. Grasping the underlying configurations, finding names, similes, and metaphors to identify with and words to express the ambiguous representations increases the parents' understanding of the ways in which these unconscious inside stories from the past are being unwittingly enacted – avoided or voided – in the current parent-baby encounter. Articulation of early subjective experience in turn reduces the tendency to bypass nonverbal experience through activity, unconscious manipulative pressures, or psychosomatic expression. Finally, such self-understanding increases parental acceptance of their own ambivalence and intuitive knowledge of the complex, subjective feelings of the baby in their care, through an empathic recognition of that baby as a separate person, sharing a similar range of emotions to themselves.

Womb, Cradle, and Couch

Of course, therapists each have their own share of mental representations which affect their practice. Like parents with their baby, each therapist approaches a client with a particular orientation that is rooted in the theoretical framework she or he holds. And so the flow of this book has come full circle; that is, I am suggesting that like parental orientations, psychoanalytic theories of developmental processes affect not only conceptualization of the patient's infancy, but of the therapy required as well. Furthermore, some parallels exist between the model of parenting described in this book, and psychoanalytic schools of thought.

Pared down to their fundamental denominators, distinctions between psychoanalytic theorists pivot on the twin axes of infantile endowment and complementary needs for care. Those theories which conceptualize the infant as basically wild, asocial, and unintegrated, will regard the care giver's task as socialization, inserting him or her into the existing social order by getting the baby to adapt. Those that regard the infant as benign and vulnerable, will emphasize the need for sensitive devotion and maternal adaptation to the baby's needs.

Broadly speaking, these are also the differing trends of early classical theorists and Ego Psychologists following Heinz Hartman and Margaret Mahler's ideas of infant adaptiveness (corresponding to the Regulator) on the one hand, and fine-tuned, empathic mothers of Object Relations theorists such as Donald Winnicott, and Kohutian Self-Psychologists (corresponding to the Facilitator) on the other. The former two regard the infant as initially undifferentiated, 'autistic', primarily narcissistic, and seeking tension release rather than company. Ascribed internal preoccupation and initial lack of discrimination mean that primary care might be shared interchangeably between mother and nanny, as, indeed, Freud conceded. In fact, in this view attachments are only gradually formed on the basis of pleasurable satisfaction of physiological needs and discharge of drive-derived excitations. Relationships are thus seen to develop from the initial state of objectlessness through what Freud called anaclitic attachments. Pathology arises as a result of *internal factors* – unresolved intrapsychic conflicts between life and death instincts (as in the Drive model) or between internecine internal urges and reality demands (as in Ego Psychology). Treatments would aim to reinforce instinct control and renunciation of drive derivatives through insight and increased ego hegemony.

However, if, as conceptualized by the Object Relations theorists such as Balint and Fairbairn, the benign baby is seen as sociable but initially in a state of merger, and undifferentiated from his or her 'selfobject' (as Self-Psychologists call it), the 'symbiotic' existence of early life will be regarded as an extension of interuterine fusion, necessitating the exclusive and constant care of the biological mother and presence of her real breast. The facilitating mother's devotion is deemed essential for future mental health, and pathology will be attributed to maternal failures, deficits, inadequate mirroring or cumulative deprivation: it is the *external environment* which is pathogenic. Psychotherapeutic treatment may aim at producing a regressive state in which archaic parental failures are rectified.

A further view is a mixture of the two above, which I referred to as bimodal. For instance, in Kernberg's early theory, and in the Kleinian framework *a priori* knowledge of the mother is coupled with innate aggression, and pathology arises from a preponderance of constitutional sadism and derivative fantasies, as well as depriving and frustrating internalized bad objects.

It seems to me that despite individual variations, in recent years psychoanalysts among the British Independents and North American Self-Psychologists, as well as contemporary psychoanalysts of other schools scattered throughout the world, now follow an interactional model of development, which resembles what I have called the Reciprocator parent. These emphasize not fusion, but what Colwyn Trevarthen termed 'intersubjectivity' – acknowledging the baby as interpersonally motivated, reality-oriented and self-regulating from the start.

In general, psychoanalysts sharing these views would, like Daniel Stern, see the innate capacities of the infant as activated in the context of responsive interaction between particular primary care givers and a particular baby, and the unfolding of these capacities as largely dependent on environmental provision of reciprocally intermeshing emotions. Above all, the infant is regarded not as a passive recipient but an active initiator, seeking a 'shareability' of interests and actions; thus, the infant is a nego-tiating contributor to the organization of the early experience, through which self and other representations are structured. The therapeutic corollary recognizes the specificity of interaction be-tween a particular analyst and particular analysand, regarding psychoanalytic process as their reciprocal construction of a real-ity of meanings.

Given this broad variety of visions, we may wonder, how is it that each psychoanalytic school of thought 'sees' a different baby? After pondering this puzzle myself, I have concluded that although these theories are based on actual observation, the per-ception of each observer is primed by the theory they hold. We each are looking at the same baby, but focusing on *different states of alertness*. As with parents whose unconscious represen-tations of the baby during pregnancy set the scene for assigning meaning to infant behaviour according to the attributes they have ascribed – benign, vulnerable, weak, demanding, powerful, vicious – so inferences made by professionals about fantasy con-tent and psychic activity are coloured by their own particular developmental model of the mind.

Caregiving is not easy. We are fallible and make mistakes. There is always a mythical analyst or parent whose perfection we fail to achieve. But we can only each be ourselves – knowing our weaknesses, building on our strengths, we can try to avoid re-peating errors by understanding rather than burying them. We are none of us one unified monolithic personality but have many voices and a mixture of emotional narratives within; recognizing this ongoing internal diversity not only enriches our own re-sources but increases receptivity to the fluidity of our own memoires and to the flow of stories inside others.

| *Epilogue*

'. . . I would love you to see him,' writes Gabriella some months after our last meeting. 'You've been so much a part of all this – conception, pregnancy, birth, and all the rest. I can certainly now understand how women keep quiet about the awful bits – you forget them, they fade, they seem so transient. Was I ever pregnant?

The passion I feel for Benjamin still amazes me; I have never loved any one person so unreservedly and unconditionally. I worry that it will overwhelm him or I will restrain him. In my worst moments I worry something will happen to him; I can't bear the desolation that envelops me when I think like that. Such a reality would be unthinkable.

Benjamin changes my perspective – I try and see the world as he sees it. For him each day is a big adventure. He expresses his pleasure so clearly, . . . I could go on (and on) . . . How my mother-in-law regards the fact that I do things differently as a direct attack on how she did things. How Jacob is so much more in love with his son than he thought he would be. How I want to get to the top but I want to be there for Ben and if I can't do that all the time, at least be not too tired to have fun when I *am* there. I want him to only be happy, to protect him from all troubles yet I want him to live life. Nothing seems as important as Benjamin.

The luxury at work is that I can gush – in limited quantities – whereas I am sure that Jacob can't. However, it's interesting how bosses who were so sympathetic during pregnancy now pretend that nothing has changed. Other people must feel this magic when they have children. Isn't it sad that we're supposed to be so cool and calm and collected and pretend it is all as before. I feel part of a club, but it's a quiet one. When the women get together at least we can all share it, but the men so often seem to be peripheral. For all my anxieties about my career I will keep them all rather than give up a second of my special relationship.

I hope we have a chance to meet again. You gave me so much – a broad perspective, coping strategies, freedom to be and a place where I could be just me with my womb, fears and joys . . .'

Appendix – Vulnerability During Childbearing

Timely therapy benefits people unable to contend with reactivation of previous traumatizing experiences or current emotional overload. Working through troubling issues and precursors of bonding disturbances during pregnancy can pre-empt parental dysfunction and forestall costly treatment of established conditions. The following chart offers guidelines to overlapping risk factors in women susceptible to distress.

Risk Indicators

Conflicted Pregnancies
- unplanned;
- untimely (too young, old, early, late);
- 'wrong' mother, father, baby;
- acute ambivalence;
- bipolar conflicts of extreme Facilitator/Regulator;
- psychosomatic discharge.

Emotional Sensitization
- post-infertility pregnancy (AIH/AID, IVF, GIFT, ovum donation);
- family history of perintatal complications;
- borderline disorders;
- neurotic defences;
- psychiatric history.

Complicated Pregnancies
- physical condition of the mother (multiple pregnancies, substance and fetal abuse, eating disorders, HIV positive, illness, disability);
- life events (bereavement, eviction, miscarriages);
- socio-economic factors (poverty, housing, unemployment);
- lack of emotional support.

Conflicted Pregnancies

Unplanned pregnancies involve moral and ethical dilemmas as to whether and how the pregnancy may be aborted or incorporated into the body of the woman or the couple's psychosocial life. When an unplanned pregnancy forces an emotional crisis within the partners' relationship, urgent counselling may be required to avert a precipitous split, or to prompt an overdue decision to separate.

Untimely pregnancies highlight unreadiness for a baby. A woman might feel that conception has come too early or too late in a relationship, or too soon after a failed pregnancy or an unmourned bereavement. Unconscious motivation to fill a gap often conflicts with realistic constraints and emotional lag.

The woman may feel she is too young or emotionally immature. Teenage pregnancies seem to be on the increase, partly due to disillusionment, misuse or lack of contraception. Various studies cite early experiences of loss, separation from primary care givers, and a high incidence of parental divorce or death in families of pregnant adolescents. Other studies attribute pregnancy to rebelliousness, loneliness, and poor self-image, finding these girls to have less secure relationships with their mothers compared with sexually active peers who do not become pregnant. However, recent Western statistics indicate that for every two adolescents who go on to have a baby, at least one aborts, possibly motivated by the realization of the difficulties involved in the precocious assumption of maternal responsibilities.

As in other conflicted pregnancies, couple therapy, to relieve some of the strains while strengthening and enriching the bond between adolescent partners, or individual therapy during pregnancy can accelerate maturation. In the case of adolescent mothers, professional support and guidance will probably continue to be needed after the birth. (A successful model of intervention in crossgenerational maladaptive parenting among adolescents was pioneered by Selma Fraiberg in San Francisco. Another, 'Genesis', operates in Boulden, Colorado.)

When the woman feels too old, or that conception has come too late to save a failing marriage, or that it is out of phase with her career, she may be in conflict about aborting this last-chance pregnancy, despite its untimeliness and risks. (This reality-bound ambivalence is to be differentiated from both long-standing phobic avoidance of pregnancy, and the manic stance of a woman whose determination to conceive late in life reflects an omnipotent desire to challenge menopause and deny mid-life awareness of mortality.) In addition to her own anxiety about the increased risks of complications, an older woman may have to contend with her family's shocked reaction, or adolescent children's embarrassment at her autumnal pregnancy. Older primagravidas may be torn between the dictates of the biological clock and demands of a profession. Others who have worked long and hard towards this conception – which these days could be the result of ovum donation in a post-menopausal woman – may be surprised by the physical toll.

While older women have rich stocks of life experience and resources of worldly wisdom to draw upon, parenthood in mid-life involves a radical shift in settled lifestyle and relationships. Although in itself not sufficient cause for psychological disturbance, coupled with the re-triggering of repressed conflicts and difficulties during pregnancy, the introduction of a baby – particularly into a mixed stepfamily – may engender generational and blood-relation realignments which destabilize family relationships. The woman, partners, or whole family may benefit from crisis intervention or ongoing help.

A 'wrong' pregnancy, in which one member of the generative triangle is felt to be at fault, constitutes a subgroup of negatively experienced pregnancies. The mother may lack confidence in herself or be considered by others to be unsuitable for mothering for a variety of realistic or imagined reasons. Daughters of depriving, intrusive, or neglectful parents, and victims of rape, incest, or abuse of any kind are all vulnerable during pregnancy to anxieties that their insides and creative nurturing capacities may have been affected. Physical experiences of having an intruder in her inner-most bodily space, the invasiveness of internal examinations, and fears of the physical experience of birth may all revive the shocked hurt and outrage of a repressed or recalled initial trauma.

When the baby's father is felt to be 'wrong', the basis may be an Oedipal fantasy or the reality that he is unloved; a donor; a seducer or rapist; a total stranger; a substitute for someone else; extramarital; or incestuous. The common denominator is that his contribution to her baby feels distasteful, forbidden or alien. An inability to overcome her 'allergic response' or 'immunological rejection' endangers the fetus with psychological or physical expulsion during pregnancy and alienation postnatally.

The 'wrong' baby may be the result of any of the above, or the 'wrong' sex, imagined or known. In cases where 'wrong' equals abnormal as revealed by tests necessitating a decision whether to undergo an abortion, both expectant parents or the woman alone may benefit from the opportunity offered by brief psychotherapy to work through crucial feelings at this critical point. In the very short time available to them, decision-making is often hampered by the confusing mixture of emotional conflicts, practical factors, ethical or religious considerations, as well as anger, irrational guilt, and in the case of prenatal tests, trepidation about incorrect diagnosis and uncertain outcome. Sometimes a baby is *psychologically wrong* – deemed to be an inadequate replacement for a previous loss, poor reparation for an aborted or dead baby, imbued with an aspect of the self that cannot be tolerated, or simply the wrong sex. For some women pregnancy arouses *acute ambivalence*, anxiety, distress, panic reactions and heightened somatic complaints, ranging from difficulties in bearing her own pregnant body and/or its contents, to intolerance about becoming a mother. Finding herself inhabiting a maternal body with an inside which, like her pregnant mother's, contains a being who has crossed the body-boundary, and will cross it again to make an exit, she may become blankly detached, disempowered or panicky and paralyzed: feeling unable to put a stop to the process and unable to sit back and watch it unfold. Others resort to extreme Facilitator/Regulator reactions.

Fetal abuse during pregnancy may necessitate urgent crisis intervention, brief therapy, or counselling, particularly when the woman or her baby are in danger. Mediation may be required to resolve internal conflicts possibly leading to habitual abortion, suicidal attempts, violence, or rejection. As noted throughout this book, ambivalence around conception has a variety of conscious and unconscious sources. Within a couple, impregnation may constitute an act of vengeance on a treacherous woman or a belittling man, and possession of his child inside her may form a means of magical control or power, changing the balance of a relationship. Where conception is motivated by pathological or perverse unconscious factors, ongoing therapy can facilitate exploration of unconscious issues and avert abusive use of the baby as sacrificial scapegoat, a transitional object, or messianic saviour. Repeated miscarriages or self-induced abortions may be overdetermined, affected by unconscious identifications, for instance with the archaic mother perceived as murderous. In some cases, revenge or rebellious proof of autonomy from the mother, and/or punishment for incestuous wishes may take the form of physical assault on the fetus, linked with child abuse. Early detection is important, and intervention as appropriate with prenatal psychotherapy, followed by infant-centred maternal supportive counselling, or psychoanalytic psychotherapy, which aim to alter negative maternal projections.

Psychosomatic discharge may be used as a means of bypassing thought, using the body to foreclose or avoid disturbing feelings. Pregnancy may be a means of denying emptiness, emotional barreness, or separateness. Conception may provide a sense of aliveness or proof of not being dead. It may compensate for loss, frustration, or deprivation, or constitute a concrete addition to the internal world. It may signify a physical return to the internal mother's womb; concrete reparation or bodily reincarnation as her mother; or an attack on the internalized maternal body now identified with her own.

Psychosomatic aggravation of common symptoms of pregnancy may become incapacitating, including excessive nausea and vomiting, choking, fatigue, asthmatic reactions, twitchings, sweating, skin allergies, digestive disorders, tension headaches, palpitations, and vague aches and pains. In my clinical experience, hysterical symptoms and dissociations in pregnancy seem to belong to that archaic class of disturbances that Joyce McDougall refers to as having a pre-symbolic psychological meaning. Paradoxically, these concrete enactments are the result of a primitive attempt to deal with intense anxieties that go unrecognized because they have been 'ejected' from consciousness since the anxieties aroused have been unable to achieve mental representation in a symbolic, verbal (i.e. thinkable) form. Couvade symptoms in expectant fathers may be of the same preverbal order.

Lack of awareness of psychological pain, and resistance to using symbolic representation and language rather than physical symptoms or hypochondriasis, creates a difficulty in using psychotherapy to treat people who have a tendency towards psychosomatic solutions. However, the distress afforded by their symptoms, and the pressure to obtain help before the birth may facilitate mental engagement. If untreated in expectant mothers, there is a danger of premature birth, feeding difficulties, and excessive somatization of the relationship with the baby.

Emotional Sensitization

Post-infertility pregnancies are often so precious that they become overvalued and vigilantly monitored, with fears that even fleeting lapses of concentration may bring about a loss. Diagnosis of infertility and prolonged treatment in themselves have cumulative effects of 'erosion of self-esteem; invasion of the couple's sexual intimacy and of her/his body; and debilitating cycles of hope, anxiety, and despair (see my 1986a, 1992a papers).

Conception following medical intervention such as GIFT, IUF or IVF introduce a third person into the intimate sexual dyad, with related Oedipal fantasies, anxieties, and sexual difficulties. In cases of gamete donation, artificial insemination, or ovum by donor, there is a fourth person: the unknown donor. Fantasies about the 'real' parent abound.

Asymmetry of their genetic relation to the baby may necessitate therapy to enable the partners to redress the emotional balance between themselves, and to deal with unvoiced recriminations, derision, shame, guilt, and pity for the infertile partner. On a deeper level, the experience of conception that bypasses identification with the fertile generative parents may also bring about oscillation between unconscious omnipotence at having circumvented parental prohibitions and fantasies of Oedipal triumph, and the underlying despair at an inability to conceive unaided as proof of internal damage and retaliation by an envious internal parent. Abrupt transition from long-standing subfertility to potential parenthood – and in some cases multiple births – impels rapid revisions of identity and internal configurations again benefiting from therapeutic help.

Individual or joint psychoanalytic psychotherapeutic treatment will have to encompass the partners' psycho-histories; their relationship; the impact of infertility; psychological residues from the long periods of invasive treatment; fears for the child's normality – given the 'abnormality' or artificiality of his or her conception; fantasies about the unknown biological parent/s ('bad blood', 'family romance'); the place of this fantasy child in their internal worlds; and issues of social secrecy relating to how much or whether to tell relatives and the child about his/her origins.

In cases of multiple conception, selective abortion may be undertaken with attendant guilt and worries about the physical and psychological effects on the remaining fetus(es), and how the choice was made. Surrogacy is a relatively rare but complex phenomenon and, like mothers giving up their babies for adoption, both the birth mother and in some cases the couple would benefit from therapeutic help if amenable to it.

Family history of perinatal complications heightens a fear of hubris: the pregnant woman may unconsciously feel unentitled to a live baby or a straightforward birth, which may draw her into re-enactments of disastrous (hearsay) labours or unconsciously selected features of these family myths. Timely therapy can release the woman from the grip of the past, enabling her to relinquish losses, and to differentiate this baby and her own pregnancy from others.

Women who have experienced an unresolved abortion, late miscarriage, stillbirth, or neonatal loss will be particularly vulnerable during pregnancy. Pregnancy often revives the grief yet blocks the mourning process. Grief may be inhibited by a magical belief in reincarnation of the dead baby in the live fetus, or a denial of the unmourned loss. In some cases, pregnancy curtails mourning, or in itself may constitute a defence against bereavement for a previous loss. The replacement child (see Sabbadini) may have to bear the brunt of unconscious aggression, maternal preoccupation with the dead, verbalized, or unspoken resentment, irrational accusations, and unresolved feelings surrounding the inadequately mourned loss during pregnancy. However, postponed mourning can be resumed, even many years after the pregnancy.

Borderline disorders are exacerbated during pregnancy by psychological vulnerability, rapid physiological changes, re-evaluation of body image, confusion of body boundaries (two people inhabiting one skin), and fluctuating shifts of identity. Insecurities are further intensified by violated gender boundaries with the tangible 'bisexual' pregnancy.

Clear-cut distinctions between inside and out, past and present, real and unreal become blurred through the permeability of internal boundaries between conscious thought, dreams, daydreams, and unconscious fantasies. This confusion is augmented by the reawakening of archaic memories, the breakthrough of unintegrated affect states, or unprocessed early experiences. Heightened sensory experience of a primitive unverbalized nature (see Ogden), modes of irrational thinking, bodily communication, and disturbingly undisguised dream images can further undermine psychic equilibrium in pregnancy.

Neurotic defences are often intensified with the threatened breakthrough of dangerous emotions and reactivation of traumatic experiences during pregnancy, and studies have found an increased frequency of neurotic and minor psychiatric disorders. What I have observed in clinical practice with neurotic women seen before conception and/or between pregnancies are periodic flare-ups during pregnancy of anxiety manifesting in panic disorders; intolerable apprehensiveness; insomnia; breathlessness; low stress tolerance; and chronic tension and irritability; likewise, the emotional disequilibrium described throughout this book, with re-evaluative disturbance of seemingly resolved issues.

As with all hypochondriacal reactions, somatic complaints may also be a call for help. However, during pregnancy they may be masked and treated as part and parcel of the physical condition, while the psycho-neurotic element is overlooked. In some women or their partners extreme defensive measures may be employed to counteract the disorganizing effects of emotional upheavals and 'bipolar' conflicts during pregnancy, such as superstitious activities, and driven, addictive, or compulsive behaviours. Paranoia and phobias, eating disorders, depression and excessive tearfulness may all manifest in greater intensity during pregnancy, and benefit from immediate psychotherapy.

Conversely, some neurotic complaints 'disappear' during pregnancy as the woman gains assurance and self-esteem. In some women conception resolves acute conflicts of femininity or sexuality and difficulties in the external relationship to her mother in which the neurotic insecurity was imbedded. Although the underpinning dynamics may remain unexplored, relief may persist uneventfully into the early years of motherhood, masked by attention being shifted on to the baby and mothering. Neurotic conflicts may flare up again in subsequent pregnancies, corresponding to a particular sibling in her family of origin, life events, or related stresses and strains in her social environment.

Despite a history of psychiatric disorder, the parents may remain well throughout pregnancy and after. Others may relapse with the life event of pregnancy, their schizophrenic delusions or hallucinations now reflecting or denying the pregnancy, with attendant risks. Affective disorders too may be focused around pregnancy, with clinical depression relating to current impoverishment and unsuitability as a future parent, and in manic states glorification of pregnancy, self, or the fetus. One to two per 1000 people suffer puerperal psychosis, including women with no previous psychiatric history, and their partners. Recent studies in England have shown that the rate of psychotic illnesses in partners of hospitalized psychiatrically ill new mothers has been found both to have more life-time and current psychiatric disorder than spouses of well women, and is associated too with marital difficulties and poor relationship with the man's own father (see Lovestone). Clinically I have found that for women who have been ill following a past birth, the undeniable physical stress and psychological upheavals of pregnancy may seem very frightening, as they spend the entire pregnancy dreading recurrence of a psychotic episode, and feel constantly scrutinized by concerned relatives and doctors. McNeil in several retrospective studies found that patients with an early postpartum onset of cycloid or affective psychosis have been less angry, more idealistic, more tense, anxious and, above all, animated or excited during pregnancy.

The etiology of puerperal psychosis is unclear, although about half the women also have non-puerperal episodes of psychosis and/or a family history of mental illness; however, it also occurs in women who had seemed healthy previously. Prognosis for recovery is excellent, but fifty per cent relapse with subsequent babies. Treatment varies. Group or individual therapy or supportive couple counselling during the pregnancy can lessen anxiety and increase adaptation to pregnancy, while working through issues of ambivalence related to becoming a parent or incorporating another child into the family constellation.

Psychoanalytic psychotherapy after the psychosis has abated can help an insightful woman to incorporate the bewildering episode into her life, and may serve a preventative function in relation to future births. An acute reaction involving schizophrenic features often requires hospitalization. Postnatally, joint admission can be arranged for mother and baby or the family. In some special units, such as the Cassel Hospital in London, a psychoanalytic approach is offered and/or family therapy may be available on an inpatient basis with outpatient follow-up. Other mother-baby units offer various types of supervised care or day hospital treatment with nursery provision.

In all cases of puerperal psychosis, confusion is a worry, and where paranoid, sexual, or hypochondriacal delusions relate to the pregnancy or baby, surveillance may be necessary to prevent the woman attempting to harm the baby through physical assault or invasive measures. There may be some difficulty containing florid symptoms in mania, as lithium crosses the placental barrier and is contraindicated during early pregnancy. It appears to be also conveyed in breastmilk: bottle feeding is usually recommended, although breastfeeding may be possible if serum levels are monitored in the mother. Neuroleptic drugs for controlling schizophrenia are considered to be safe.

Complicated Pregnancies

Physical conditions due to chronic illness during pregnancy, or pregnancy-related conditions which necessitate hospitalization or bedrest at home, immobilize the woman during an already difficult period and add to the burden of anxieties about the effects of her illness on the fetus, other children, and her partner. Where there is a sense of herself and/or the fetus being bad for each other (placental insufficiency, Rhesus incompatibility, and so on), prenatal bonding may be affected by worries about exacerbation of her own condition due to the pregnancy, and guilt, resentment, and tension caused by simultaneously wanting to retain the pregnancy yet release them both from their mutual bondage.

Disabled women may find pregnancy a particularly rewarding time, as it grants creative and effective use of their bodies, and offers a rare opportunity to be accepted on equal terms by other women sharing the same female experience. However, a disabled woman may become sadly disillusioned as dire warnings, medical or parental disapproval, and prejudicial comments mount as she becomes more visible and self-determining. At times she may find herself ostracized as the embodiment of her pregnant peers' fears of a deformed baby.

Sadly, HIV infections are becoming an increasing problem during pregnancy. In therapeutic treatment, it is useful to differentiate between three groups of women:

- those who discover themselves or their partners to be HIV-positive during pregnancy and have to face the repercussions of this diagnosis for themselves as well as for their babies;
- those who are HIV-positive and discover themselves to be pregnant, having then to make a decision whether to carry to term and face the risk of infecting the infant, or to abort;
- those who knowingly have decided to become pregnant, although or because, they or the partner are HIV-positive.

The current view is that pregnant women who are themselves ill are potential carriers, and children born to seropositive mothers are almost ten times more at risk than those born to infected mothers who are well. In addition to having to contend with fears for the future and social isolation or rejection, there is a long period of uncertainty about the infant's state (up to twenty-four months a toddler born to an infected mother may show positive results due to maternal antibodies). Maternal anxieties also focus on their own health (current research suggests that pregnancy may accelerate the condition in women whose immune systems have been damaged), and ability to nurture the child while themselves feeling ill. Like other minority groups, her plight may be made more difficult through prejudice and stigmatizing, even by health care workers.

Substance abuse during pregnancy may be a continuation of a previous addiction, or directly related to imminent motherhood. Briefly, in the latter cases, drugs, alcohol excess, eating disorders, or even smoking may constitute a test of endurance to prove the baby's durability, or an attempt by the mother to compensate for putting up with being pregnant, or a need to replenish resources depleted by the 'parasitical' fetus (see Chapter 3).

Negative socio-economic factors and life events such as bereavement, eviction, or redundancy constitute a double burden of adjustment in a woman already preoccupied with the demands of pregnancy. Screening and positive test results generate much anxiety, and even if a woman is determined not to abort the malformed baby, she will benefit from counselling or psychotherapy that enables her to work through her guilt, sense of failure, and ambivalent feelings towards the child before the birth, and to prepare for the ordeal ahead. Support may be needed postnatally.

Lack of emotional support constitutes perhaps the most significant factor in a woman's vulnerability to the stresses of pregnancy and motherhood. Women who are in an unsatisfying or damaging relationship need support and possible couple therapy to explore whether the situation can be improved before the baby is exposed to the stresses of parental discord, or whether separation might be preferable. Women who find themselves alone following death, divorce, or desertion during pregnancy are particularly susceptible to depression, and unlike women who have chosen to become single mothers, may be unable to contemplate a future as a sole parent. As stated earlier, mourning is often delayed and self-esteem distorted by the emotional processes of pregnancy and childbearing.

For all women with inadequate emotional support, the experience of care in psychotherapy might be their first encounter with benevolent mothering. Internalized, it can mitigate some of the negative emotional experiences of their lives, and serve as a model for mothering the baby. Most probably already affecting their current relationships, unrealistic inside stories impede realistic attachment to the baby, whether they involve childhood traumata, unmourned losses, unrelinquished past grievances, or the inability to establish a fruitful sense of agentic self-hood.

The aim of dynamic psychotherapy or psychoanalysis is to relieve psychic pain and to help people resolve internal 'fixations' and repetitive conflicts which prevent them approaching new situations in a fresh and flexible manner. Internal changes occur through emotional reactivation of unconscious archaic experiences in the present, and projection of unconscious internal representations on to the analyst or therapist. Ideally, curiosity, self-expression, and the search for meaning give the impetus for continuing self-reflection even after symptomatic discomfort has subsided, enabling the person to gradually internalize the function of psychoanalysis, metabolizing and working through difficulties as they arise. As such therapy releases resources which have been occupied in defensive manoeuvres of dispersal, hiving-off, deflection, or silencing interval voices. Thus enriched by self-acceptance, vulnerable people find greater trust in their capacities to meet challenges of love and hate with the ambivalent means at their disposal.

| Bibliography

Balint, M. 1965. *Primary Love and Psycho-Analytic Technique.* Liveright.

Bassen, C. 1988. 'The impact of the analyst's pregnancy on the course of analysis', *Psychoanalytic Inquiry* 8:280–298.

Benson, P. *et al.* 1987. 'Foetal heart rate and maternal emotional state', *British Journal of Medical Psychology* 60:151–154.

Benedek, T. 1970. 'The psychobiology of pregnancy', in *Parenthood – its Psychology and Psychopathology.* Eds A. J. Anthony and T. Benedek, Little Brown.

Bibring, G. 1959. 'Some considerations of the psychological processes in pregnancy'. *Psychoanalytic Study of the Child* 16:9.

Bion, W. 1962. *Learning from Experience.* Heinemann.
— 1970. *Attention and Interpretation.* Maresfield.

Bollas, C. 1987. *The Shadow of the Object: Psychoanalysis of the Unthought Thought.* Free Association Books.

Bourne, S. and Lewis, E. 1992. *Psychological Aspects of Stillbirth and Neonatal Death,* an annotated bibliography. Tavistock Publications.

Bowlby, J. 1950. *Maternal Care and Mental Health.* WHO Publications.
— 1979. *The Making and Breaking of Affectionate Bonds.* Tavistock Publications.

Chamberlain, D. 1987. 'The cognitive newborn: a scientific update', *British Journal of Psychotherapy* 4:30–69.

Coltart, N. 1988. 'Diagnosis and suitability for psychoanalytical psychotherapy', *British Journal of Psychotherapy* 4:127–134.

Cowan, P. and C. 1992. *When Partners Become Parents.* Harper Collins.

Daws, D. 1989. *Through the Night: helping parents and sleepless infants.* Free Association Books.

DeCasper, A. J. and Fifer, W. P. 1980. 'Of human bonding: newborns prefer their mother's voices', *Science* 208, 1174–7.

Deutsch, H. 1944. *The Psychology of Women: a psychoanalytic interpretation.* Grune & Stratton.

Eliot, T. S. 1963. *Collected Poems 1909–1962.* Faber and Faber.

Etchegoyen, A. 1993. 'The analyst's pregnancy and its consequences on her work', *International Journal of Psycho-Analysis* 74:141–150.

Fairbairn, W. R. D. 1952. *An Object-relations Theory of the Personality*. Basic Books.

'Fels Study': Crandall, V. 1972. *Seminars in Psychiatry* 4: 383–307.

Fenster, S. 1983. *The Therapist's Pregnancy: intrusion in the analytic space*. Analytic Press.

Fonagy, P., Steele, H. and Steele, M. 1991. 'Maternal representations of attachment during pregnancy predict the organization of infant-mother attachment at one year of age', *Child Development* 62:981–905.

Fraiberg, S. 1980. *Clinical Studies in Infant Mental Health: the first year of life*. Tavistock Publications.

— 1987. 'The adolescent mother and her infant', in *Selected Writings of Selma Fraiberg*. Ohio University Press.

Freud, A. 1966. *Normality and Pathology in Childhood*. Hogarth Press.

Freud, S. 1901. *The psychopathology of everyday life*, Vol. VI SE, Hogarth Press.

— 1909. ['Little Hans'] *Analysis of a phobia in a five-year-old boy*, Vol. X SE, Hogarth Press.

— 1915. *The unconscious*, Vol. XIV SE, Hogarth Press.

— 1918. ['Wolf Man'] *From the history of an infantile unconscious* Vol. XVII SE, Hogarth Press.

'Genesis': Community Infant Project, Mental Health Centre, Boulder, Colorado.

Gerzi, S. and Berman, E. 1981. 'Emotional reactions of expectant fathers to their wives' first pregnancy', *British Journal of Medical Psychology* 54: 259–265.

Gottlieb, S. 1989. 'The pregnant therapist: a potent transference stimulus', *British Journal of Psychotherapy* 5:287–299.

Greenberg, M. 1985. *The Birth of a Father*. Continuum.

Heimann, P. 1989. *About Children and Children No-Longer: Collected papers 1942–1980*. Ed. M. Tonnesman. Routledge.

Hartman, H. 1958. *Ego Psychology and the Problem of Adaptation*. International Universities Press.

Herzog, J. M. 1982. 'Patterns of expectant fatherhood', in *Father and Child: developmental and clinical perspectives*. Eds S.H. Cath, A. R. Gurwit and J. M. Ross. Little, Brown.

Hey, V. *et al.* 1989. *Hidden Loss: miscarriage and ectopic pregnancy.* The Women's Press.

Holden, J. M., Sagovsky, R. and Cox, J. L. 1989. 'Counselling in a general practice setting: controlled study of health visitors' intervention in treatment of postnatal depression', *British Medical Journal* 298: 223–226.

Jaques, E. 1955. 'Socialsystems as a defence against persecutory and depressive anxiety', in *New Directions in Psycho-Analysis.* Eds M. Klein, P. Heimann and R. E. Money-Kyrle. Tavistock Publications.

Joyce, J. 1922. *Ulysses* (1947). Van Leer.

Jung, C. G. 1963. *Memories, Dreams and Reflections.* Routledge.

Kernberg, O. 1980. *Internal World and External Reality: object relations theory applied.* Aaronson.

Kestenberg, J. 1976. 'Regression and reintegration in pregnancy', *Journal of the American Psychoanalytical Association* 24: 213–250.

Klein, M. 1952. 'Some theoretical conclusions regarding the emotional life of the infant', in *Envy and Gratitude and Other Works* (1984). Hogarth Press.

— 1958. 'On the development of mental functioning', in *Envy and Gratitude and Other Works* (1984). Hogarth Press.

Lax, R. 1969. 'Some considerations about transference and countertransference manifestations evoked by the analyst's pregnancy', *International Journal of Psycho-Analysis* 50: 363–372.

Layland, R. 1981. 'In search of a loving father', *International Journal of Psycho-Analysis* 62: 215–224.

Leverton, T. L. and Elliott, S. A. 1989. 'Transition to parenthood groups: a preventive intervention for postnatal depression', in *The Free Woman: Women's Health in the 1990s.* Eds E. V. Van Hall and W. Everaerd. Parthenon Press.

Liley, A. W. 1972. 'The foetus as a personality', *Australian and New Zealand Psychiatry* 6:99.

Lovestone, S. and Kumar, R. 1993. 'Postnatal psychiatric illness: the impact on spouses', *British Journal of Psychiatry* 163: 210–216.

Mahler, M., Pinke, F. and Begman, A. 1975. *The Psychological Birth of the Human Infant.* Hutchinson.

Mariotto, P. 1993. 'The analyst's pregnancy: the patient, the analyst, and the space of the unknown', *International Journal of Psycho-Analysis* 74:151–164.

McDougall, J. 1989. *Theatres of the Body*. Free Association Books.

McNeil, T. E. 1988. 'A prospective study of postpartum psychosis in a high-risk group', *Acta Psychiatrica Scandinavia* 77: 604–610.

Morley, P. 1992. 'On fatherhood', *Esquire* April.

Nadelson, C. *et al*. 1974. 'The pregnant therapist', *American Journal of Psychiatry* 131:1107–1111.

Niemela, P. 1992. 'Vicissitudes of mother's hate', in *Of Mice and Women: aspects of female aggression*, Academic Press.

Oakley, A., McPherson, A. and Roberts, H. 1990. *Miscarriage*. Penguin.

Ogden, T. 1989. *The Primitive Edge of Experience*. Jason Aaronson.

Penn, L. 1986. 'The pregnant therapist: transference and countertransference issues', in *Psychoanalysis and Women: contemporary reappraisals*. Ed. J. L. Alpert. Analytic Press.

Pines, D. 1972. 'Pregnancy and motherhood: interaction between fantasy and reality', *British Journal of Medical Psychology* 45: 333–343.

Piontelli, A. 1992. *From Fetus to Child: an observational and psychoanalytic study*. Routledge.

Raphael-Leff, J. 1983. 'Facilitators and Regulators: two approaches to mothering', *British Journal of Medical Psychology* 56: 379–390.

— 1985a. 'Facilitators and Regulators: vulnerability to postnatal distress', *Journal of Psychosomatic Observations and Gynaecology*. 4: 151–168.

— 1986a. 'Infertility: diagnosis or life sentence?', *British Journal of Sexual Medicine*. 3: 28–29.

— 1986b. 'Facilitators and Regulators: conscious and unconscious processes in pregnancy and early motherhood', *British Journal of Medical Psychology* 56: 379–390.

— 1989. 'Where the wild things are', *International Journal of Pre- and Perinatal Studies* 1: 78–89.

— 1991a. *Psychological Processes of Childbearing*. Chapman & Hall.

— 1991b. 'Psychotherapy and pregnancy', *Journal of Reproductive and Infant Psychology* 8: 119–135.

— 1991c. 'The mother as container: placental process and inner space', *Feminism and Psychology* 1: 393–408.

— 1992a. 'The Baby-Makers: psychological sequelae of

technological intervention for fertility', *British Journal of Psychotherapy* 7: 239–294.

— 1992b. 'Reproductive life – impact of medical intervention: "In sorrow shalt thou bring forth" ', in *Reproductive Life: advances in research in psychosomatic obstetrics and gynaecology*. Eds K. Wijma and B. von Schoultz. Parthenon Press.

— 1992c. 'When eternals change: invited commentary on reproductive issues and the National Health Service', *APP Psychoanalytic Psychotherapy Newsletter* Summer.

— 1992d. 'Transition to parenthood – Infertility: creating a family', in *Infertility and Adoption*. Eds D. Reich and J. Burnell. Adoption Centre Publications.

Rayner, E. 1990. *The Independent Mind in British Psychoanalysis*. Free Association Books.

Robson, K. and Kumar, C. 1980. 'Delayed onset of maternal affection after childbirth', *British Journal of Psychiatry* 136: 347–353.

Rosenblatt, J. *et al.* 1962. 'Progress in the study of maternal behaviour in the rat: hormonal, nonhormonal, sensory and developmental aspects', *Advances in the Study of Behaviour* 10: 226.

Ross, J. M. 1975. 'The development of paternal identity: a critical review of the literature on nurturance and generativity in men', *Journal of the American Psychoanalytic Association* 23: 783–818.

Rossetti, D. G. 1870. 'Pandora', in D. Panofsky, *Pandora's Box* (1978). Princeton University Press.

Sabbadini, A. 1988. 'The replacement child', *Contemporary Psychoanalysis* 24:528–547.

Salk, L. 1973. 'The role of the hearbeat in the relations between mother and infant', *Scientific American* 220: 24–29.

Samuels, A. 1989. *The Plural Psyche: personality, morality and the father*. Routledge.

Savage, W. 1984. 'Sexual intercourse during pregnancy and fetal distress', *British Journal of Sexual Medicine* 11.

Stern, D. 1985. *The Interpersonal World of the Infant: a view from psychoanalysis and developmental psychology*. Basic Books.

Tolstaya, S. 1863. *The Diaries of Sofia Tolstaya* (1985). Jonathan Cape.

Trevarthen, C. 1979. 'Instincts for human understanding and for cultural cooperation: their development in infancy', in *Human Ethology: claims and limits of a new discipline*. Eds von Cranach *et al*. Cambridge University Press.

Winnicott, D. W. 1951. 'Transitional objects and transitional phenomena', in *Through Paediatrics to Psycho-Analysis* (1975), Hogarth Press.

— 1954. 'Metapsychological and clinical aspects of regression within the psycho-analytical set-up', in *Through Paediatrics to Psycho-Analysis* (1975), Hogarth Press.

— 1956. 'Primary maternal preoccupation', in *Through Paediatrics to Psycho-Analysis* (1975), Hogarth Press.

— 1957. *The Child and the Family*. Tavistock Publications.

— 1974. *Playing and Reality*. Penguin.

| *Index*